Foreword

The English National Board is delighted to publish this report as part of its series: *'Researching Professional Education'*.

The aim of this series is to make the results and implications of research commissioned by the Board readily available to the key stakeholders: to policy makers, managers, practitioners, researchers and educationalists. The Board recognises that it is important for these groups to have ready access to relevant research findings from which to plan and implement developments in nursing, midwifery and health visiting education.

The Board's research and development programme is planned to ensure that education for practice is relevant both professionally and academically. Research-based evidence therefore provides an important dimension for policy development.

This research is based on a comprehensive literature review of nursing's contribution to rehabilitation within primary and secondary care and the multi-professional team and an analysis of curriculum documentation relating to pre- and post-registration education.

The outcomes of the research include discussion of:

● the need to articulate clearly the nurse's role in rehabilitation

● the dimensions of an expanded role in rehabilitation

● the need to address the existential, biographical and temporal dimensions of rehabilitation.

The report forms the first phase of a major study into the nurse's role in rehabilitation. An empirical study is currently being commissioned to explore the nurse's role in rehabilitation. The Board will consider the findings from both research projects in relation to policy developments.

Professor Ron De Witt

Chairman, English National Board

Professor Jeff Thompson

Chair, Research and Development Group, English National Board

London, 1997

Contents

1.	**Context and Method**	**6**
1.1	Setting the scene	6
1.2	Method	10
1.3	Project management	14
1.4	Language	16
2.	**Rehabilitation and Nursing: An Overview**	**18**
2.1	Rehabilitation: a service in flux	18
2.2	The nurse's role in rehabilitation: current perspectives	20
3.	**Rehabilitation: Establishing the Dimensions**	**25**
3.1	Rehabilitation: a concept looking for a definition	25
3.2	The ICIDH: a stimulus for change	29
3.3	Biopsychosocial and temporal models of disability and rehabilitation	31
4.	**Rehabilitation: Important Components**	**35**
4.1	Patient involvement and empowerment	35
4.2	Incorporating the perspectives of the disabled person	36
4.3	The involvement of family carers	40
4.4	Team-working: fulfilling the reborn certainty	43
4.5	Rehabilitation: neglected areas in the literature	45
5.	**Narrowing the Focus: From Models to Mid-range Theories and Concepts**	**48**
5.1	Identifying recurring themes	48
5.2	Stress/coping and related concepts	48
5.3	Motivation	51
5.4	Psychosocial interventions	52
6.	**Rehabilitation: Identifying the Dimensions of the Nurse's Contribution**	**56**
6.1	Rethinking rehabilitation	56
6.2	Beyond physical care	58
6.3	Towards a more extensive contribution	61
6.4	Expanding the nursing role	61
6.5	Constructing a framework	66

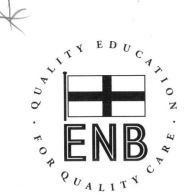

RE
PRO
EDU

*A series from the English National Board
for Nursing, Midwifery and Health Visiting*

New Directions in Rehabilitation: exploring the nursing contribution

Mike Nolan

Andrew Booth

Janet Nolan

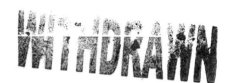

University of Sheffield

London, 1997

Published by

The English National Board for Nursing, Midwifery and Health Visiting,
Victory House, 170 Tottenham Court Road, London W1P 0HA
Telephone: 0171 388 3131
Fax: 0171 383 4031
E-mail: enb.link@easynet.co.uk
www site: http://www.enb.org.uk

© English National Board for Nursing, Midwifery and Health Visiting, 1997

ISBN 1 901697 08 8

This report has been prepared for publication by
Jill Rogers Associates, Cambridgeshire
Design by Sadler, Suffolk
Printed by Chiltern Press, Luton

Acknowledgements

The project team would like to extend their sincere thanks to a number of people, without whom this report would not have been possible, and to all the institutions who forwarded copies of their curricula. Members of the Steering Group provided help and advice and were always insightful and supportive; our thanks in particular to Sonia Crow for her perseverance and forebearance.

Thanks also to members of the library staff throughout the university, but particularly Susan Paisley, Jane Harrison and Nicola Howson at ScHARR. Finally, there is one individual who is owed a particular debt of gratitude and for whom the words 'above and beyond the call of duty' take on new meaning; Helen Mason, without whose input this document would never have emerged. Diolwch yn Fawr Helen.

The Project Team

Mike Nolan, Professor of Gerontological Nursing, University of Sheffield

Andrew Booth, Director of Information Resources, School of Health and Related Research, University of Sheffield

Janet Nolan, Lecturer in Nursing, University of Sheffield

The Steering Group

Millie Carter, Nursing Officer, Department of Health

Sonia Crow, Assistant Director for Educational Policy (Research and Development), English National Board for Nursing, Midwifery and Health Visiting

Christine Fessey, Education Policy Officer, English National Board for Nursing, Midwifery and Health Visiting

Jane Marr, Education Officer, English National Board for Nursing, Midwifery and Health Visiting

Pat Noons, Nursing Officer, Department of Health

David Thompson, Director of Research and Development, School of Nursing, Faculty of Health, University of Hull (Chair)

Karen Waters, Professor of Nursing, School of Nursing, Midwifery and Health Visiting, University of Manchester

Biographical details of the authors

Mike Nolan is Professor of Gerontological Nursing at the University of Sheffield. Over the last 15 years he has been actively involved in addressing the needs of older people and their carers as a practitioner, educator and researcher. Mike is committed to narrowing the theory-practice gap and has published widely in a range of academic and professional journals. He has particular interests in family caregiving, chronic illness and disability and the development of better services for individuals with ongoing health care needs.

Andrew Booth is Director of Information Resources at the School of Health and Related Research (ScHARR), University of Sheffield. He has worked in a variety of health settings over the last 14 years, the most recent being at the King's Fund as Information Services Manager. Andrew has a specific interest in all aspects of evidence-based practice and has published widely on the topic. His expertise lies in finding the evidence and in advising on different literature review methodologies.

Janet Nolan is a Lecturer in Nursing at the University of Sheffield. She has considerable experience of nurse education at all levels, having taught on a wide range of pre- and post-registration courses from Certificates to Masters degrees. She has also been involved in the design and implementation of curricula across a similarly diverse spectrum of courses. She has particular interest in the development of specialist practice roles in community settings, and is currently course leader BMedSci (Hons) Specialist Community Nursing and Health Care Practice.

7. **Towards a Broader Conceptualisation**   **69**

    7.1   Testing the framework   69

    7.2   Rehabilitation: contrasting models   70

8. **Preparing for a More Active Role**   **78**

    8.1   Knowledge and skills for practice   78

    8.2   Specific model or eclectic knowledge base?   79

9. **Conclusions: Realising the Potential**   **85**

    9.1   The nursing role   85

    9.2   What is rehabilitation?   86

    9.3   Opportunities and barriers   86

    9.4   Organisation of care   90

    9.5   Nurse education   91

References   **93**

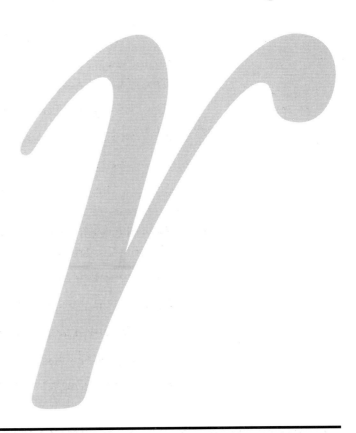

CONTEXT AND METHOD

1.1 Setting the scene

Against a background of sustained and increasing change in the organisation and delivery of the health service, the English National Board for Nursing, Midwifery and Health Visiting (the Board) commissioned a series of projects concerned with preparation for multiprofessional and multiagency health care. This report presents the results of a literature review investigating the nursing contribution to rehabilitation within the multidisciplinary team.

The original requirement was to undertake a comprehensive literature review of nursing's contribution to rehabilitation within primary and secondary care and the multiprofessional team. The second stage of the project consisted of analysing curriculum documentation relating to pre- and post-registration education. The curriculum analysis determined the extent to which the course content, teaching and learning strategies promote the knowledge and skills to enable the nurse to make a positive contribution to rehabilitation within the multiprofessional team in primary and secondary health care settings. The results of the curriculum analysis are not included in this report, but can be found in the other, fuller account of the project (Nolan et al, 1997). The four specific client groups included in the review are:

- the older adult

- the disabled young adult

- those who have experienced major trauma

- those who have experienced coronary heart disease, stroke or other pathologies emerging from the literature.

The review aims to advise the Board of the implications for pre- and post-registration education and to inform validation and monitoring processes.

The project team believed that the rapidly changing nature of health care and the lack of consensus as to what constitutes rehabilitation meant a traditional systematic review would be inadequate, and likely to reinforce the *'sterile empiricism and compartmentalisation'* characterising much current thinking (Swift, 1989). The review process was therefore built upon the belief that progress is unlikely unless there is a widening of conceptual horizons and a willingness to look constructively and critically at the available literature and the assumptions underpinning current practice.

Preliminary examination of the literature suggested that rehabilitation is dominated by a biomedical and functional model which fails adequately to account for the views of disabled or ill people and their carers. Consequently, policy development has been limited, primarily because policy-makers have little idea of the key issues (Corbin and Strauss, 1988; Beardshaw, 1988). Lazarus (1992) argues for a more contextual and process-orientated approach to end the current *'professional deception'*. It was therefore considered essential to extend the review to include the perspectives of disabled or chronically ill people and their carers, requiring that *temporal* and *biographical* dimensions be incorporated.

It was necessary to consider the influence of these decisions on the review process in general and the sampling of databases in particular. The review excluded children, people with mental health problems and those with learning difficulties and focused on the four client groups (the older adult, the disabled young adult, those who have experienced major trauma, and those who have experienced coronary heart disease, stroke or other pathologies emerging from the literature). However, even with this restricted focus, a preliminary scan of the databases suggested there were more than 5,000 relevant references. It was well beyond available resources to include all these in the review, so it was decided to undertake a conceptual synthesis of key themes in the rehabilitation literature, together with a carefully targeted review and analysis of curriculum documents in selected domains. This required a strategy and sampling rationale which could be justified on theoretical grounds; Rolland's model (1994) was selected for this purpose. Rolland describes a biopsychosocial typology of chronic illness which, he asserts, provides a comprehensive *'landscape'* of illness and disability which differentiates conditions on criteria of particular importance for interventions regarding onset, course, incapacity and outcome. Using this typology as a basis, a sampling frame for the review was generated as follows:

1.1.1   Potentially fatal conditions

a.   Acute onset/constant course: stroke and myocardial infarction (MI)

b.   Gradual onset, relapsing course: multiple sclerosis (MS)

1.1.2   Generally non-fatal conditions

a.   Acute onset/constant course: spinal injury

b.   Gradual onset/progressive course: arthritis

These conditions were sampled across all care settings and references dealing with the needs of family carers were included. Using this strategy it was anticipated that the four client groups, which had been identified by the Board, would be addressed. Stroke and MI are among the most frequent causes of chronic illness and disability; stroke is mainly associated with the older adult, whereas MI often occurs in younger people. Multiple sclerosis not only affects a generally younger age group but runs an unpredictable and highly variable course. Spinal injury on the other hand is usually associated with major trauma, is unpredictable and unexpected and often involves younger adults. Arthritis (rheumatoid and osteo) constitutes a diverse group of conditions affecting younger and older adults, are usually non-fatal and run a gradual but progressive and unpredictable course.

Completing the review therefore presented logistic and conceptual challenges which required careful consideration, as the decisions made would inevitably affect the end result. Beardshaw (1988) argues that there are several *'vexed problems'* concerning the purpose and future of rehabilitation, mainly arising from the narrow perspectives that have traditionally been applied. As the preliminary work began, a number of paradoxes and contradictions emerged which substantiated Beardshaw's arguments; the literature is long on rhetoric but practice lags some way behind:

- The literature extols the benefits of holistic rehabilitation, but in practice the dominant focus is on functional ability with psychological, social and other needs receiving scant attention.

- While the greatest demands for rehabilitation come from those with chronic and progressive illnesses, who have ongoing needs, rehabilitation is usually seen as a finite process, as the emphasis on outcome measurement confirms.

- The importance of patient and carer participation and empowerment are stressed, yet most assessment criteria applied in practice are objective, and the subjective perceptions of patients and carers are often overlooked.

Furthermore, many key elements of rehabilitation, such as team-working, quality of life and even the notion of rehabilitation itself, lack conceptual clarity and have varied meanings and interpretations depending on the theoretical orientation used. Compounding such difficulties, some areas of rehabilitation use a number of models, whereas in others there is a dearth of good conceptual work.

Related issues arise with respect to the nurse's role in rehabilitation. Some argue that there is a rehabilitative component to the nurse's role in virtually all areas of practice, while others advocate a specialist role in defined areas. This is an important distinction which suggests either the need for a generic approach that permeates education at pre- and post-registration levels or alternatively casts rehabilitation mainly within the post-registration domain. Conversely, both approaches might be appropriate, with generic competencies that can be applied across contexts being developed prior to qualification, but which require modification, perhaps by condition or by illness stage, at post-registration level.

Another problem was posed by the fact that, as Beardshaw (1988) contends, most debates on rehabilitation, including those concerned with the nurse's role, are confined largely to the medical or paramedical literature which, while extensive, provides a restricted perspective. The wider sociological and other literature offers valuable insights which may enhance practice and policy. However, integrating this literature is a considerable task and potentially raises fundamental questions about rehabilitation in general and the nurse's role in particular.

Faced with the above tensions there were two main options for the analysis of the references obtained. The first was to undertake a traditional review, identifying current rehabilitation practice and the nurse's role within the multidisciplinary team. This would have provided a framework for the subsequent curriculum analysis but was likely to prove a rather sterile exercise, largely confirming what has already been identified by others – that, particularly in the UK, the nurse's role in rehabilitation is limited and under-developed (Waters, 1991; 1996; Walker, 1995).

A second option was to attempt something more creative but less safe and certain. Based on the premise that the current theoretical underpinning of rehabilitation practice generally fails to address a number of key issues, particularly the existential, biographical, temporal and relational impact of chronic illness and disability, it is possible to construct a case for what the nurse's role in rehabilitation *might* be if broader parameters were applied. It was considered that this provided a more useful alternative.

Having taken this decision, and because of the tensions between a generic as opposed to a specialist role in rehabilitation, it was considered necessary to conduct two, initially separate, analyses. It was decided therefore both to describe the nurse's *actual* (i.e. current) role in rehabilitation and, based on analyses of the generic literature, to attempt to develop a framework for a *potential* role. Subsequently, the literature pertaining to the nurse's rehabilitative role in the identified conditions was used as a *partial test* for the models' adequacy and comprehensiveness. In this way it was hoped that an expanded or modified generic model might emerge or alternatively a generic model together with one or more complementary or alternative models relevant to the differing conditions.

This process is seen as being equivalent to an empirical investigation using a grounded theory methodology. Consistent with the tenets of this approach the review avoided an *a priori* definition of rehabilitation, identifying instead a broad range of literature sources considered to provide an informed opinion. Data analysis similarly avoided pre-determined categories but adopted a three-phase approach in which each reference was summarised and subjected to content analysis. As major themes were identified within each source, constant comparison was undertaken across sources so that the boundaries and parameters of themes could be explored. The resultant synthesis was 'grounded' in the data and what emerged can be considered broadly equivalent to a 'grounded theory' of rehabilitation and the nurse's role within it. Once basic themes emerge it is usual to adopt a theoretical sampling approach to further study, whereby subsequent informants (literature sources) are selected purposively to reflect key aspects of the developing theory. This is to determine if 'saturation' has been reached.

Morse (1994) argues that all qualitative research follows four essential phases, albeit with differing emphasis depending on the approach utilised:

- comprehending

- synthesising

- theorising

- recontextualising.

Comprehension is said to have been reached when '*the researcher has enough data to write a complete, detailed, coherent and rich description'*. Synthesising then involves the '*merging of several stories, experiences or cases to describe a typical, composite pattern'*. Theorising is '*a process of development in which the "best fit" data is achieved by constructing alternative formulations until the most comprehensive, coherent and simple model is found'*. However, Morse considers that recontextualising is the '*real power'* of qualitative research as it involves further elaborating the emerging theory so that it is applicable to other contexts of interest. Such a logic was also applied to the review process.

The initial review, in providing an overall description of the elements of rehabilitation and the nurse's role within it, equates with the stage of early theorising. Saturation from the general literature had been reached at the end of the initial stages, resulting in an embryonic framework suggesting the relationship between key components of rehabilitation. It was then necessary to subject this framework to critical scrutiny to determine if it could be 'recontextualised' to other relevant settings. To achieve this, a theoretical sample was adopted reflecting a number of dimensions of chronic illness; this was the purpose of Rolland's biopsychosocial typology (1988; 1994).

While it would have been possible to adopt a different sampling method which may have given other results, the project team believe the method used was robust and comprehensive given the parameters of the commission and the resources available.

In terms of the curriculum analysis the intention was to use data provided by the Board relating to current course provision for the selected conditions and DipHE pre-registration programmes of education, and to subject a random sample of curriculum documents to a detailed analysis.

Resulting from these conceptual and methodological decisions, the four aims of the study were identified as:

- To undertake a synthesis of current definitions and concepts and models of rehabilitation to identify major themes and their implications for the development of the nursing role and the educational preparation for that role.

- To undertake a comprehensive literature review in selected areas which, taken together, cover the major domains of chronic illness and disability.

- To select a random sample of curriculum documentation for existing courses relevant to the conditions reviewed and analyse these in terms of content and teaching and assessment methods.

- To provide a report to the Board which would assist in the process of developing the nurse's contribution to rehabilitation in an informed and innovative way.

Early discussions with the Steering Group resulted in modification and extension of these aims to an expanded range of courses which, while not condition-specific, might be expected to have a rehabilitative component, e.g. course 941 – Caring for Older People, and specialist community courses.

Only a brief summary of the detailed results of the curriculum analysis and separate reviews of the specific conditions is provided here. The primary intention of this report is to consider the nurse's role in rehabilitation and to present a model of the rehabilitation process in general and a framework for an expanded nursing role. Readers requiring further details of the curriculum analysis and separate reviews are referred to Nolan et al (1997).

1.2 Method

1.2.1 Rationale underpinning the search and literature review

A clear understanding of the philosophy and methods of this review is necessary to consider its findings. It was acknowledged that the potential to identify future directions for the nursing contribution would be compromised by an *a priori* definition of 'rehabilitation'. This review aimed to provide a conceptual synthesis of rehabilitation, as well as a more detailed analysis of the five aspects of rehabilitative care selected.

The review employed established techniques from the social sciences where *'the review of the literature involves the identification of a cluster of ideas from which critical elements are distinguished, conceptualised, and linked as an organised statement on the existing body of knowledge...'* (Helmericks et al, 1991). The sampling frames for a number of thematic literature searches are the bibliographic lists which 'map' significant contributions to the topic. A cumulative approach is used across multiple databases until repetition of materials occurs and further exploration provides nothing new.

The need for a thematic approach was identified when more than 2,000 references on rehabilitation published in nursing journals were retrieved from a single database (CINAHL, 1982-1995). From this, an estimated total of over 5,000 articles was projected, and the total was likely to be substantially larger if topics such as multidisciplinary working were included. Such a large-scale analysis was beyond the constraints of the project team, particularly as the Board had identified specific issues of concern that merited more detailed analysis, such as *nursing roles* and the organisation of *multidisciplinary teams*. Moreover, the project team was keen to challenge the medical model of rehabilitation by reviewing studies representing patients' views of rehabilitation. It was felt, therefore, that the literature review would best be served by a two-phase approach focusing first on the concept of rehabilitation followed by an exploration of its manifestations within the specified conditions.

The appropriateness of the above approach is best illustrated by contrast with the quantitative systematic overview, currently promoted by groups such as the Cochrane Collaboration. Guidance provided at Cochrane Collaboration Review Protocol Writing Workshops (Oxman, 1994) emphasises the importance of defining the following parameters before embarking on the review process:

- population

- intervention

- outcome

- study design.

Analysis of the above parameters within the context of this study revealed the inappropriateness of a 'Cochrane-like' approach. Our study design incorporates a heterogenous *population* achieved by selecting conditions of differing degrees which present and develop differently. It also covers contrasting likelihoods of fatality and markedly different age profiles. Consideration of *intervention* is similarly heterogeneous, with the concept analysis aiming to identify a full range of possible interventions including physical, psychological and social, as well as the explicitly holistic. Clearly it is contrary to the study aims arbitrarily to define rehabilitation and only to consider studies meeting predetermined criteria, or to blur the distinction between the constituents of rehabilitation by treating it as a single intervention. In the latter case, critical appraisal of the Cochrane Collaboration review on stroke rehabilitation units (Langhorne et al, 1993) often focuses on the lack of clarity with regard to interventions performed in such units.

In the context of *outcome*, with conditions of such disparate onset and course it would be difficult to specify an optimal period for follow-up. Also, easily measured outcomes such as mortality are inappropriate to this study – again this is a reported deficiency of the Cochrane Collaboration stroke rehabilitation units review. Finally, although it is useful to draw on evidence of rigorous *study design* if available, the range of methodological approaches necessitated by the foci of our study, including concern with patient views, precludes basing our conclusions exclusively on such sources.

However, it is felt that the validity of the literature search is enhanced by adopting three principles from the *systematic* literature review – that it should be *systematic*, *explicit* and *reproducible* (Booth, 1996). The following sections document this process and provide supporting detail on the management of the literature review component of the project.

1.2.2 Identification and selection of studies

A major feature of this project is the wide variety of sources consulted (Barber, 1995). Separate searches were performed for the six facets of the study. This has resulted in some duplication between references because of subject overlap, but was felt to be of value in assuring the completeness of subject coverage and in cross-validating search strategies. A more significant practical problem is in overlap between databases. Although bibliographic management software usually enables duplicate checking, this primarily eliminates duplicates from related sources (e.g. Social Science Citation Index and Science Citation Index) and does not help to manage, for example, the estimated 35% overlap between MEDLINE and EMBASE (Burnham and Shearer, 1993). Of a total of 5,358 references 1,114 (21%) were removed due to cross-database duplication.

The major databases used were CINAHL, for its nursing and rehabilitation emphasis, and MEDLINE and EMBASE for their coverage of general and physical medicine. It was recognised, however, that exclusive use of CINAHL and MEDLINE, though recommended for nursing topics (Brazier and Begley, 1996), could lead to a North American bias, so the Nursing and Midwifery Index (University of Bournemouth) and the AMED (British Library) were also searched. The theoretical component of the first phase of the review also suggested the use of the Social Science Citation Index and the Science Citation Index, while the emphasis on organisation of the delivery of care was appropriate to HEALTHSTAR (formerly HEALTHPLAN). The databases of the Nuffield Institute for Health (HELMIS), Department of Health (DHSS-DATA) and the King's Fund Library Catalogue were also used, but yielded little additional material to that identified from the other databases or through following up references from retrieved articles or other published lists. During the second phase of the study, the appearance of the Cochrane Library, with access to the Cochrane Collaboration Register of

Clinical Trials, containing more than 100,000 studies, and the Database of Abstracts of Reviews of Effectiveness (DARE), provided the opportunity to identify the evidence base around rehabilitation for the target conditions. Finally, coverage of basic rehabilitation texts was provided through a search of the US National Library of Medicine book catalogue from 1990 onwards. All searches were confined to the English language and performed across varying time periods according to the coverage of individual databases (Table 1.1).

AMED	1985-1995
CINAHL	1982-1995
Cochrane Library	1960s-1995
DHSS-DATA	1983-1995
EMBASE	1980-1995
HELMIS	1984-1995
King's Fund Library	1992-1995
Nursing and Midwifery Index	1994-1995
Science Citation Index	1981-1995
Social Science Citation Index	1981-1995

Table 1.1: Time periods searched among individual databases

Coverage of the specific conditions focused on the last 10 years (1986-1995), whereas coverage of work on the theories and models of rehabilitation aimed to be more far-reaching and broad-ranging, and each database was searched from its date of inception.

1.2.3   Phase 1: theories and models of rehabilitation

Search strategy

In the first of the two phases of the literature review, appropriate search terms were identified by conducting trial searches in the databases and inspecting both thesaurus and naturally-occurring terms in initially-retrieved relevant items. These were then applied in the full search procedure. This approach occasionally yielded important terms that were inadequately covered by assigned indexing terms. For example, the concept of 'social support' had no corresponding index term, yet figured significantly in the literature. Text searches (of titles and abstracts) were therefore used to complement index term searches to improve sensitivity of coverage. The concept of rehabilitation was searched for at the broadest possible level; on MEDLINE, for example, this included the subject term *rehabilitation* exploded to include narrower terms from the subject hierarchy, truncated as a textword and truncated in either the source field (e.g. journals containing rehabilitation in their title) or the institutional address field. The search strategy for phase 1 of the project aimed to narrow these very broad subsets in order to identify:

- general overviews of rehabilitation with special reference to the role of the nurse and of multidisciplinary teams

- discussions of theoretical frameworks and models for rehabilitation both general and in relation to specific rehabilitation contexts.

The former approach uses a variant of the Cochrane Collaboration search strategy (Lefebvre, 1994) to identify reviews, and thus utilises text searches of terms such as *overview, review* and *meta-analysis,* as well as publication types where assigned. However, the multidisciplinary team is a central concept that might yield additional materials though not necessarily in reviews, so the terms *multidisciplinary* and *team* were thus used in isolation and together.

A very sensitive strategy was used in search of articles on the theoretical base of rehabilitation, in order to identify as many as possible with any relevance to the project. Terms used included *model* and *theory* as well as the subheading *classification* and other related textwords such as *concept* and *definition*. Preliminary filtering was necessary to exclude 'false drops' occurring in connection with animal models of disease. Since there was a dearth of articles specifically covering models of rehabilitation, this aspect of the search was broadened to include *theoretical models of chronic disease*.

Results

Approximately 900 unique references were identified from the journal databases and a further 130 monographs and textbooks were identified from the National Library of Medicine Book Catalogue. Of the combined references, 163 (approximately 15%) were considered, on the basis of titles and abstracts, worthy of more detailed examination. Major reasons for excluding studies included instances where references were reviews of case reports, discussions about the coding of conditions, or reviews of very specific physical rehabilitation interventions; in cases of doubt about an article's possible value the full text was obtained. In addition to the computerised search the main reviewer (MN) also adopted a 'snowball strategy' of references cited frequently in the articles reviewed.

1.2.4 Phase 2: the target conditions

Search strategy

The rehabilitation of any one of the target conditions might constitute a full-scale literature review in its own right, so in an attempt to improve specificity and keep the review process manageable it was decided that conditions would be accessed only through assigned subject terms, such as *myocardial infarction* or *cerebrovascular disorders* (stroke) and not through free-text variants. Where the structure of the database permits (e.g. MEDLINE and HEALTHSTAR), articles were restricted to those where the condition is a major focus of an article. Although it was decided not to limit retrieval of articles to specific study designs considered to be dominant in a hierarchy of evidence (e.g. randomised controlled trials or meta-analyses) publication types such as correspondence or editorials were excluded. Finally and most importantly, the emphasis in retrieving items was on those covering:

● the work of multidisciplinary teams

● nursing aspects and nursing roles

● patient perspectives, including psychosocial factors.

The activities of multidisciplinary teams within each condition were searched for independently of a specific mention of rehabilitation, using *multidisciplinary* and/or *team*. It was felt that the retrieval of extraneous materials was a small price to pay for a full understanding of the multidisciplinary team dynamic. In fact the number of articles specifically addressing the team role in rehabilitation was disappointingly low.

The retrieval of relevant condition-specific articles with a nursing component was addressed in one of two ways. In databases that were non-specific to nursing (e.g. HEALTHSTAR, EMBASE and the Citation Indexes) the sensitive strategy *nursing* was used to pick up all occurrences of terms such as *nurse, nurses* and *nursing* in conjunction with rehabilitation of the specific conditions. In the remaining databases with a specific nursing remit (such as MEDLINE and CINAHL) *all articles* from the Nursing Journals Subset dealing with rehabilitation of the specific conditions were retrieved together with *any articles* from the remainder of the database retrieved using the sensitive *nursing* strategy.

Articles dealing with the patient's perspective were retrieved through a number of complementary approaches such as using the *psychology* subheading (MEDLINE), the index terms *Psychosocial-Factors*, *Patient-Satisfaction* and *Nurse-Patient-Relations*, and using free-text terms including *psychosocial*, *patient attitudes* and *patient views*.

Results

Phase 2 of the literature search identified approximately 3,100 references, of which 410 (approximately 13%) merited further examination. Studies were excluded according to considerations such as only mentioning the nurse in passing, or where the activities of a professional rehabilitation nursing organisation were described. Particular importance was attached to descriptions of the patient experience of a condition, with a focus on rehabilitation. However, there appear to be few systematic attempts to survey patients' perceptions and a large proportion of anecdotal experiences. Table 1.2 shows the number of items retrieved against those subsequently obtained for each condition.

Condition [subject terms]	No. of items retrieved	No. of items obtained	% of items obtained
Stroke [cerebrovascular-disorders]	866	120	14%
Myocardial Infarction [myocardial-infarction]	494	86	17%
Spinal Injuries [spinal-injury] [spinal-cord-injury]	503	72	14%
Arthritis [explode arthritis]	832	62	7%
Multiple Sclerosis [multiple-sclerosis]	426	70	16%

Table 1.2: Items retrieved and obtained for the target conditions

1.3   Project management

As already stated, it was neither possible nor desirable for this project to tackle its subject matter in the manner of a quantitative systematic literature review. Nevertheless it *has* been useful to follow the stages of project management outlined in the NHS Centre for Reviews and Dissemination (1996) guidelines on conducting a review. These stages, as manifest in this particular project, are outlined in Table 1.3.

Stage 0	Identification of the need for the review
Stage 1	Background research and problem specification
Stage 2	Requirements of the review protocol
Stage 3	Literature searching and study retrieval
Stage 4	Assessment of studies for inclusion on basis of relevance and design
Stage 5	Assessing the validity of the studies
Stage 6	Data extraction
Stage 7	Data synthesis
Stage 8	Structure of the report
Stage 9	Review of report for scientific quality, content and relevance
Stage 10	Submission of report and plans for dissemination

Table 1.3: Stages of the project

In conducting what have, in fact, been six separate reviews relating to the five specific conditions and the concept of rehabilitation itself, an iterative process (corresponding to stage 3 of the above) has been followed by the project team:

a.   Literature searching

b.   Loading of references to a reference management database

c.   Elimination of duplicates

d.   Production of a master list for each topic

e.   Identification of relevant articles

f.   Generation of document requests

g.   Identification of document locations

h.   Requesting of documents

i.   Receipt of documents

j.   Logging of documents on reference management database

It is important to document that while literature searching and obtaining of articles are typically costed in bids for large-scale reviews, it is essential not to overlook these other, less apparent, but nevertheless heavily labour intensive stages. For example in the present project it was calculated that 15-20 minutes was spent acquiring and recording *each* article: since 573 references were obtained, even applying the more conservative estimate, the search process required 143 hours (4.1 working weeks) of clerical input, in addition to searching of databases.

Once references were obtained they were subject to detailed analysis, undertaken in two phases. The first phase considered the generic literature on rehabilitation and the second, the condition-specific elements. The analysis strategy consisted of three stages. Stage one involved reading the references and compiling notes on their content. These notes were analysed to isolate the main themes, a number of which emerged, for example:

•   definitions of rehabilitation

•   outcomes of rehabilitation

•   models of rehabilitation

•   the nurse's role in rehabilitation

- frequently appearing concepts e.g. powerlessness, helplessness

- patient involvement

- carer involvement

- team working.

In the second phase the original notes were condensed and grouped theoretically under general headings as indicated above.

The third phase comprised a synthesis of these themes to determine their parameters and major components and to cross reference these conceptually to identify areas of similarity and contrast; this provided the basis for the construction of the initial framework for the nurse's role in rehabilitation.

An identical process was followed in reviewing the five conditions, and each review was used to help 'recontextualise' the initial framework. Subsequently the results from all the reviews were brought together in a form of 'meta-synthesis' to produce the contrasting *'restricted'* and *'comprehensive'* models of rehabilitation and a framework for identifying the dimensions of the nursing role (see Chapters 6 and 7).

1.4   Language

Before presenting the results of the review it is necessary to consider briefly how chronic illness and disability are characterised. The use of language in this area raises a number of delicate and contested issues. Verbrugge and Jette (1994) argue that a *'bedlam vocabulary'* exists in which words and phrases have been invented without their meaning being made explicit; clarity is missing even with respect to the meanings of rehabilitation, chronic illness and disability. Many writers do not attempt a definition and either use the terms synonymously or talk of 'chronic illness and disability' as automatically linked concepts. Most authors who do define disability use the World Health Organisation's International Classification of Impairment, Disability and Handicap (ICIDH, WHO, 1980); however, even this is not universally accepted. There are numerous definitions of chronic illness but again no apparent consensus. However, Miller (1992a) argues that two generalities underlie most definitions of chronic illness: they affect more than one, and often multiple, aspects of the mind, body or spirit systems, and the demands of the illness are never completely eliminated. This reinforces the need to adopt a longitudinal and temporal perspective. A definition of chronic illness is therefore not provided in this review but the above premises are accepted.

More recently Baker et al (1997) talk of *'people living with disabilities and unstable and progressive conditions'*, highlighting the dynamic and interactive nature of these conditions, and for a full understanding of rehabilitation, it is important to reflect this dynamic. Adding a further layer of complexity, those advocating a social model of disability (e.g. Oliver, 1993) argue that rather than people having a disability, they are *'dis-abled'* by a society which does not adequately acknowledge and cater for their needs. Once again consensus as to the meaning of terms is absent but consistency is required. For the purposes of this review the authors adopted the term chronically ill and disabled people.

The following chapters present the findings of the literature review and the emerging models of rehabilitation. Chapter 2 provides an overview of rehabilitation services and the nurse's current role, while Chapter 3 establishes the dimensions within which rehabilitation might be considered. Chapter 4 discusses important concepts relating to rehabilitation, and Chapter 5 looks at theories and concepts related to rehabilitation. Chapter 6 presents potential developments for the nursing role, and a suggested framework for beginning such developments;

Chapter 7 discusses one of the themes identified in Chapter 6 in relation to the five conditions included in the specific reviews and presents two contrasting models of rehabilitation. Chapter 8 considers the knowledge base underpinning an expanded nursing role, Chapter 9 presents conclusions emerging from the project.

REHABILITATION AND NURSING: AN OVERVIEW

2.1   Rehabilitation: a service in flux

According to Dutton (1995) the origins of modern rehabilitation date back to the early 1800s, but as others point out, the two World Wars brought the concept to prominence (Blaxter, 1976; RCP, 1986; Walley, 1986; Beardshaw, 1988; Becker and Kaufman, 1988; Waters, 1991). During this period rehabilitation was primarily associated with younger people (Becker and Kaufman, 1988; Mulley, 1994), the main intention being to restore them to a state of fitness so that they might return to battle or to productive employment (Blaxter, 1976; Ward and McIntosh, 1993; Mulley, 1994). However, over the last 50 years rehabilitation has been influenced by a number of factors which have both extended its scope and greatly increased the number of professional groups who claim an active role in the process.

Symington (1994) identifies seven *'megatrends'* which he considers to have shaped current practice in rehabilitation:

- the changing demography of illness and disability, particularly the rise in chronic diseases

- the emancipation of disabled people

- a shift in policy from isolating disabled people from the wider community through to their segregation and hopefully final integration

- shifts in service delivery from institutional to community settings and the emergence in most countries of rehabilitation as a distinct specialty

- concerns over the rising costs of health care in general and rehabilitation in particular with a resultant focus on efficiency and effectiveness

- the development of 'assistive technology' ranging from simple aids to complex information systems

- the shift from empiricism to applied science and the growth of rehabilitation as a scientific discipline.

While such trends are apparent in all developed countries they are not equally influential. Some of the megatrends, for example, the emphasis on cost-effectiveness, are more pertinent in a private health care system such as that in the US, where rehabilitation is required to be *'resource wise'* (Cope and Sundance, 1995). On the other hand, the concept of rehabilitation as a distinct area of practice is underdeveloped in the UK (RCP, 1986; Waters, 1996). Despite these obvious differences Symington's framework is a useful heuristic device and highlights the dynamic and evolving nature of rehabilitation; as Mulley (1994) notes *'the concept, style and purpose of rehabilitation is changing'*.

The first of Symington's megatrends, the growth in prevalence of chronic illness, has exerted a considerable influence but is one to which health care in general, and rehabilitation in particular, has been slow to respond. While it has been recognised for some time that chronic illness and disability place the greatest demands on health services (Strauss et al, 1984; Corbin and Strauss, 1988; RCP, 1986; Anderton et al, 1989), the full extent of such demands is only now becoming apparent (Asvall, 1992; Thorne, 1993; Pollock, 1993; Symington, 1994; Toombs et al, 1995; Bowles et al, 1995), fuelled in part by the rising numbers and proportion of older people (Waters, 1991; Tallis, 1992; Radley, 1994; Mechanic, 1995a). Historically, however, the needs of chronically ill and disabled people have been poorly addressed within modern health care systems, where acute care is seen as more prestigious and important (Charmaz, 1983; Strauss et al, 1984; Waters, 1991) and the emphasis is primarily on cure (Strauss and Corbin, 1988; Waters, 1991; NOP, 1996). Consequently, most services operate a *'acute simple disease model'* (Pawlson, 1994), with a curative orientation frequently applied inappropriately to chronic illness (Pott, 1992), while services are usually delivered by health professionals educated with cure in mind (Thorne, 1993). The needs of individuals with changing and fluctuating disabilities are poorly catered for (Beardshaw, 1988) and the system generally fails to respond appropriately to chronic illness (Eubanks, 1990; Braden, 1993).

While much is written about 'holistic care', the organisational infrastructure and philosophy of health services are geared towards a clinical perspective, with the medical model providing the *'key reference point'* for current rehabilitation services (Finkelstein and Stuart, 1996). The primary focus of interventions is on disability and physical/functional improvement (Barnitt and Pomeroy, 1995) which fails to meet the needs of those with chronic illness (Strauss and Corbin, 1988). These points will be elaborated further when considering definitions and models of rehabilitation in Chapter 3.

Most people with chronic illness have *'to live with rather than die from'* their condition (Verbrugge and Jette, 1994), so existing time-limited models of health care delivery and rehabilitation are largely inadequate. This is clearly evident in the current emphasis on outcome measurement (in Chapter 3.1); as Blaxter (1976) notes, chronic illness is lifelong and it is inappropriate that rehabilitation is evaluated on the basis of a simple dichotomy (success or failure) at a given time. A major distinguishing feature of chronic illnesses is their temporal dimension (Radley, 1994; Toombs et al, 1995); in recognising this there is a need to move beyond the *'blind fight against disease'* in order better to understand how people with chronic illness experience their lives (Rijke and Rijke-de-Vries, 1992). Accepting this position means that for many individuals the aim of care is not a return to a former state but is about helping them to continue to develop personally within their illness (Milz, 1992).

Andrews (1987), citing Partridge (1980), suggests four categories of patients may benefit from rehabilitation:

- those with a localised injury who are expected to make a full recovery without multidisciplinary input

- those expected to make a full recovery but require a multidisciplinary input

- those in whom some recovery is expected, where the aim is to achieve the optimal functional improvement by the application of specific therapeutic techniques

- those with progressive and on-going conditions where more emphasis is placed on social, psychological and environmental factors than specific techniques.

The first of the above groups falls outside the scope of this review and would not be considered by most people to come under the rubric of rehabilitation. However, as this review highlights, the literature pays most attention to the second and particularly the third groups, whilst the last is the subject of considerable rhetoric but little else.

Following a major review of disability and rehabilitation services in the UK, Beardshaw (1988) highlighted the absence of an effective national system, a consequence of the failure to implement the recommendations of numerous reports spanning some 40 years, a situation also noted by others (Waters, 1991). Beardshaw described the picture as bleak and identified major inadequacies in primary and secondary care; she also warned that the situation might worsen if, in moves towards community care, the health service transferred responsibility for long-term care to other agencies. Contemporary studies of the health care received by disabled people suggests that little has improved in the last decade (NOP, 1996; Baker et al, 1997).

The recent White Paper on the future of the NHS (Secretary of State for Health, 1996a) reaffirms the basic principles on which the NHS was founded and highlights the need for it to be responsive and sensitive to patients and carers:

> '*Modern health care has increasingly focused on the* experience *of individual patients. People want to be treated with dignity and respect. They want the right to participate in discussions which affect them. They want to be supported, if possible at home or in their community – by a service which is focused on their needs.*'
> (Secretary of State for Health, 1996a p4 original emphasis)

The above, together with the increased emphasis on primary health care (Secretary of State for Health, 1996b; 1996c) means considerable opportunities are emerging to extend rehabilitation practice. Some shifts in thinking are apparent, with acknowledgement that rehabilitation has for too long focused on illness and disability at the expense of health and wellbeing (RCN, 1994) and that concepts such as health promotion are as valid for disabled people as for the able bodied (Renwick et al, 1996). However, much needs to be done before such ideals permeate practice. As Oliver (1993) notes '*all is not well in the kingdom of rehabilitation*'; a consideration of how the nurse's role in rehabilitation is currently described will help to confirm this.

2.2 The nurse's role in rehabilitation: current perspectives

In considering the nurse's current role in rehabilitation two major orientations are apparent; in one, rehabilitation is seen as a component of most nursing care, while in the other, rehabilitation fits under the general heading of 'specialist' practice. Reflecting the former orientation Henderson (1980) for example suggested that nurses are (or at least should be) '*rehabilitators par excellence*', while Waters (1987) argued that an element of rehabilitation can be discerned in a wide spectrum of nursing activity. More recently however, possibly reflecting the situation in the US and the increasing trends towards 'specialist' practice in the UK, rehabilitation nursing is portrayed as a distinct area of care. Indicative of this is the publication *Standards of Care for Rehabilitation Nursing* (RCN, 1994) the introduction to which states:

> 'Rehabilitation nurses *in the United Kingdom have been developing their role over the last few years, to the point that other professionals now recognise them as valuable members of the interdisciplinary team. With the formation of the Rehabilitation Nurses Interest Group in 1990 a commitment was made by the committee and membership to raise the profile of the rehabilitation nurse's role. One of the aims of the group was to try to come to an agreement on what the rehabilitation nurse's role entails. The production of this booklet is the first step in that process.*'
> (RCN, 1994 emphasis added)

This is instructive for a number of reasons. First, it demonstrates the emergence of a distinct form of practitioner, the 'rehabilitation nurse'. Second, despite claims that such nurses are recognised as '*valuable members of the interdisciplinary team*' there is an identified need to '*raise the profile of the rehabilitation nurse's role*'. Achieving this is likely to present quite a challenge, particularly as there is some uncertainty as to the role of such a practitioner, hence the need for the booklet.

This should come as no surprise, however; even in the US, where the rehabilitation nurse is recognised as a specialist practitioner and educational provision reflects this (Waters, 1996), there are still a number of tensions. Although some argue that the rehabilitation role is unique (Leidy et al, 1990; Burggraf and Barry, 1995), others see it as integral to nursing care in general (Henderson et al, 1995; Stryker, 1996). Moreover, even though a specialist role is fairly well-established in the US, there is evidence that:

- such a role is not valued by other groups of nurses (Purk, 1993)

- the role itself lacks clarity (Gibbons et al, 1995)

- there is inadequate educational preparation for such a role (Hermann and Bays, 1994), and many practitioners have limited experience and training (Gonthier and Habel, 1994).

Therefore, while some claim that rehabilitation nursing is a recognised specialty in the UK (Gale and Gaylard, 1996), it is still a *relative newcomer* (Johnson, 1995) and, if the US experience provides any indication, it faces a number of challenges before it establishes its credibility.

The purpose of this section is to describe the nurse's generic role in rehabilitation based on the UK literature. It is considered inappropriate to include the American literature at this point, but this will be drawn upon when reflecting upon what the nurse's role in rehabilitation *might* be.

Probably the most comprehensive study of the nurse's role in rehabilitation in the UK was undertaken by Waters (Waters, 1991; 1996; Waters and Luker, 1996). This raises a number of points helpful in setting a context against which to consider the other literature. Waters indicates that the majority of the rehabilitative effort in the UK is confined to a hospital setting and focuses on physical care, the primary purpose being to return patients to a level of independence and discharge them to the community. Patients are largely passive recipients of this process and the needs of their carers are rarely considered until discharge. Prime responsibility for rehabilitation is vested with therapists, and the nurse's role, although not unimportant, is considered secondary, comprising three main components:

- *'general maintenance'*, including both the overall management of the ward and maintaining patients' physical wellbeing by attention to personal hygiene, nutrition, skin care etc.

- *'specialist'*, where the nurse is seen to have a degree of expertise particularly in continence and skin care

- *'carry-on'*, in which the nurse maintains the progress made by therapists, especially in walking and dressing, throughout the 24-hour period.

However, Waters (1991; 1996) identifies a number of problematic areas; nurses tend to lapse into traditional practices and *'do for'* the patient rather than promoting independence. This is reinforced by the routine organisation of work, for example, early morning dressing where there is pressure to *'get things done'*. Furthermore the carry-on role is compromised by the fact that nurses often lack the requisite knowledge to assess progress and maintain the patient's skills in dressing and mobilising. Compounding this is the failure to acknowledge potential role overlap between therapists, with channels of communication being poorly developed.

Possibly the most disturbing finding, however, is Waters' conclusion (reinforced in other studies unrelated to rehabilitation) that even within the 'specialist' areas of continence promotion and skin care, nurses often treat these as a set of practical tasks and appear unaware of, or do not apply, a coherent assessment framework.

While identifying a number of factors, including limited educational preparation and a range of organisational issues, as contributing to this situation, Waters (1991) concludes that urgent attention must be paid to the whole setting of rehabilitation wards. She also believes that there is a need for more education in the field, together with the development of an appropriate model for the nurse's role in rehabilitation. Waters is rightly cautious about generalising from her small-scale study, but as she points out, a considerable gerontological literature reinforces her overall conclusions.

In stark contrast to this bleak picture, Sheppard (1994a; 1994b) recounts the establishment of a nursing development unit dedicated to the rehabilitation of elderly people. This action research study presents an insightful account of the effort, determination and inspiration required to establish a more holistic and individualised approach to rehabilitation. Underpinning the unit were a number of key principles including the need for the patient and family to be key players in the rehabilitation process, together with a nursing role primarily concerned with the phased withdrawal of physical support while simultaneously paying increased attention to emotional and psychological components of care. Implementing these principles was not easy, however, and nurses often had to convince patients that they should not be doing things for them. This necessitated the creation of explicit mechanisms, such as a patients' forum, to facilitate a more active patient role.

Tensions were also apparent in the channels of communication between various disciplines, with difficulties in ensuring continuity of care, especially between nurses on day and night duty. Sheppard describes how such challenges were addressed largely successfully and presents an optimistic picture of rehabilitation nursing as a complex area of practice which extends far beyond physical care to include the creation of a general environment in which hope can flourish. Specific interventions such as facilitating grieving and the use of music as a form of relaxation are also described.

While this study suggests untapped potential for a wider nursing role in rehabilitation, creating it will require considerable effort, commitment and perseverance. It also necessitates overcoming a number of stereotypical ideas arising not only from other disciplines but also from within nursing. There is a need for an explicit philosophy of care allied with an organisational framework in which nurses have the autonomy to act independently. However, possibly one of the greatest challenges is posed by the largely invisible and subtle nursing role described by Sheppard which *may*, as this review will highlight, struggle to gain acceptance in a health care world increasingly dominated by quantifiable outcome measurement and the logic of the randomised controlled trial. The widely contrasting accounts by Waters and Sheppard provide a useful framework and context in which to consider the remaining literature.

The fundamental problem is the failure to clarify and define the nurse's role in rehabilitation and its 'invisibility' in the wider literature. Although authors such as Henderson (1980) describe nurses as *'rehabilitators par excellence'*, and others suggest a number of roles such as: *reactivation, resocialisation* and *reintegration* (Jackson, 1984), such positive attributes are not reinforced in nursing and medical texts (Sheppard, 1994a; 1994b; Waters, 1996; Livneh, 1995; Jelles et al, 1995), and Sheppard concludes that *'nursing and nurses are notable in the literature about rehabilitation by their virtual absence'*. Walker (1995) notes that nurses are unable to define their role in rehabilitation and, as she and others have suggested, see rehabilitation largely as the domain of the therapy disciplines, particularly physiotherapists (Pollock, 1993; Walker, 1995; Johnson, 1995; Waters and Luker, 1996). This reflects the currently dominant view of rehabilitation as a largely physical process, with restoration of function being the ultimate aim (Myco, 1984; Walley, 1986; Beardshaw, 1988; Waters, 1991; 1996; Waters and Luker, 1996; Sheppard, 1994a; 1994b). Consequently, rehabilitative effort focuses primarily on the acute phase of illness/disability (Gibbon and Thompson, 1992), within a hospital setting (Walley, 1986; Waters, 1987; 1991; Waters and Luker, 1996; Walker, 1995). Moreover, the educational preparation of nurses generally pays scant regard to rehabilitation (Walley, 1986; Waters, 1987; 1991; 1996; Gibbon and Thompson, 1992; Sheppard, 1994a; 1994b) and is concerned mainly with acute care. Commentators other than nurses have noted the lack of attention given to chronic illness and suggest that this may account for nursing's failure to meet the needs of disabled people both in hospital (Beardshaw, 1988) and in their own homes (NOP, 1996).

It is perhaps not surprising, therefore, that nurses are generally given a secondary role in the rehabilitation process (Waters, 1991; 1996; Johnson, 1995; Gibbon and Thompson, 1992) comprising a number of components and underpinned by a number of assumptions; these include:

- Maintenance of patients' physical wellbeing by attention to basic care needs, such as skin, nutrition and hygiene (Andrews, 1987; Waters, 1987; 1991; 1996; Johnson, 1995). This is characterised by Johnson (1995) as having patients clean, comfortable and ready for therapy. Indeed some authors suggest that this is nursing's major contribution to rehabilitation (Baggerley et al, 1995).

- A specialist role in areas such as continence promotion and care of the skin (Waters, 1991; 1996).

- Creating and sustaining a suitable environment for rehabilitation (Jackson, 1987; Waters, 1987; 1991; 1996; Sheppard, 1994a; 1994b) which facilitates the identification of patients' motivation, hopes and aspirations and their active participation. However, despite this stated intention, patients are largely passive recipients of rehabilitation (Walley, 1986; Waters, 1987; 1991; 1996).

- Reinforcing the input of others, mainly therapists (Waters, 1991; 1996; Waters and Luker, 1996; Sheppard, 1994a; 1994b; Gibbon and Thompson, 1992; Johnson, 1995; Squires, 1996). For example Johnson (1995) sees nurses as providing the *'glue or mortar'* that holds the bricks (i.e. therapy) together.

- A 24-hour presence is often portrayed as nursing's unique contribution (Walley, 1986; Andrews, 1987; Waters, 1987; 1991; 1996; Sheppard, 1994a; 1994b), but it seems pertinent to ask what nurses *do* during this period.

On the basis of the available literature the current nursing role in rehabilitation is narrowly construed and does not reflect the more holistic model suggested by authors such as Sheppard (1994a; 1994b). Waters (1996) argues that the nurse's role in rehabilitation is, or should be, multifaceted and that what makes it unique is not its individual components but their combination. She suggests that the current emphasis on primary care provides an opportunity to reconceptualise rehabilitation and for nursing to realise its potential.

Other nursing authors, however, still paint a more 'traditional' picture in which the primary emphasis is placed on the prevention of deterioration and the restoration of functioning (Gale and Gaylard, 1996). While this is, and will certainly remain, a central part of the nurse's role, the wider focus described by Sheppard (1994a; 1994b) seems slow to permeate the professional psyche. The recent standards of care documentation on rehabilitation nursing (RCN, 1994) recognised the need to shift the emphasis away from illness and disability, towards health and wellbeing, with the aim of empowering clients. This, it is suggested, requires the application of a health promotion model to rehabilitation nursing, but it seems that achieving this will require considerable effort.

CHAPTER 2

As noted earlier, Oliver (1993) suggests that *'all is not well'* with rehabilitation and it is apparent that there is scope for considerable development of the nurse's role. There is an extensive biomedical literature on acute rehabilitation and a broader socio-psychological literature on the needs of disabled and chronically ill individuals who, it is argued, also have legitimate claims to rehabilitative care. The central premise of this review is that these literatures must be synthesised if a more complete understanding of rehabilitation generally, and the nurse's role in particular, is to emerge.

Speaking of a similarly extensive and disparate literature on family caregiving, Gubrium (1995) suggests that in such circumstances a simple literature review is inadequate, with the likely result being *'more of the same'*. He argues that a critical assessment is required which attempts to deconstruct general assumptions and return to basic questions such as *'what is this thing some call caregiving?'*. A similar logic is adopted in this analysis which reflects upon the adequacy of current models of rehabilitation practice when confronted with the literature on the experiences of disabled and chronically ill people. This is based on the belief that such an approach is essential if the current rhetoric of empowerment, participation and involvement is to be realised. Paraphrasing Gubrium (1995), therefore, the initial question to address is: 'what is this thing some call rehabilitation?'.

REHABILITATION: ESTABLISHING THE DIMENSIONS

3.1 Rehabilitation: a concept looking for a definition

Speaking of rehabilitation, Brandsma et al consider that:

'Consensus about definition of concepts is mandatory for communication, research and educational purposes. This is especially true for a concept for which a classification is developed (as for example rehabilitation).'

(Brandsma et al, 1995; p119)

Although an element of consensus is important, there is always a tension between overly precise definitions resulting in a *'premature closure of ideas'* (Kaplun, 1964), and definitions which are so inclusive as to be almost meaningless. Such tensions are apparent with respect to the definition of rehabilitation. However, definitions are important for theoretical and operational purposes and also because they exert considerable influence on resultant services (Blaxter, 1976; Oliver, 1993).

A number of authors highlight the difficulties of achieving a uniform definition of rehabilitation (Walley, 1986; RCP, 1986; Waters, 1987; 1991; 1996; Beardshaw, 1988; Tallis, 1992; Keir, 1996) and many commentators either provide no definition or assume a consensus (Waters, 1996; Waters and Luker, 1996). Consequently although the concept of rehabilitation is frequently used it is often misunderstood (RCP, 1986). To compound such difficulties many definitions are accepted either implicitly, uncritically or both. Despite considerable variation, however, it is possible to discern commonalties, at least in the literature emanating from the health disciplines such as medicine, nursing and the therapies. A few selected definitions serve to illustrate this.

In an introductory text for medical students, Garrison (1995) suggests that rehabilitation is concerned with *'the improvement of function and adjustment to disability rather than disease cure'*. Similarly, following extensive consideration of the literature Jelles et al (1995) conclude that:

'The aim of rehabilitation medicine is to help patients to reach and maintain an optimal level of everyday function and wellbeing despite the permanent presence of a disease or affection.' (p123)

The above definition is instructive because it highlights, despite claims to multidisciplinarity in rehabilitation, that the primary focus often remains on medicine and that when cure is not possible, a return to function becomes the aim. This should not necessarily be decried, however; as Evans et al (1995) contend, when cure is unobtainable, independence in the activities of daily living (ADL) is the first choice of outcome for many patients.

For some individuals, however, especially those with permanent disability, this aim may be unobtainable, and seeking independence and optimal functioning may be counter-productive. Barnard (1995) criticises the rhetoric of independence when applied to disabled people, describing autonomy as the *'worst illusion'* and self-sufficiency as the *'most destructive aim'*. Such goals are appropriate for many people but the adequacy of a definition of rehabilitation focusing primarily on functional independence, assuming this will result in wellbeing or adjustment, is questionable.

Adopting a wider perspective, Waters takes rehabilitation to mean:

'... the whole process of enabling and facilitating the restoration of a disabled person to regain optimal functioning (physically, socially and psychologically) to the level that they are able or motivated to achieve.'
(Waters, 1996 p242)

While broadening the consideration of functioning and adding a welcome element of patient self-determination, the emphasis on 'restoration' apparent in this definition might be criticised by some as focusing too much attention on previous levels of ability (Blaxter, 1976; Milz, 1992; Barnard, 1995). Although many definitions of rehabilitation include a range of outcomes in, for example, physical, mental, social, economic domains, most also emphasise restoring or returning an individual to full or optimal levels of functioning (Fairhurst, 1981; Walley, 1986; RCP, 1986; Jackson, 1987; Becker and Kaufman, 1988; Ben-Sira, 1989; Melvin, 1989; Dutton, 1995; Porter, 1995; Dejong and Sutton, 1995; Vaughan and Bhakta, 1995; Lankhorst et al, 1995). As with independence, this focus on function is an appropriate goal for some but suggests that rehabilitation ends when function is restored, ignoring the ongoing needs of those with permanent disabilities. The above definitions seem most appropriate for individuals in Partridge's (1980) second and third categories – individuals expected to make a full recovery or where some improvement is anticipated, but are less relevant for his fourth category.

Moreover despite the inclusion of a number of domains, a physical orientation towards rehabilitation still predominates, especially in hospital-based services (Waters, 1991; 1996; Keith and Lipsey, 1993; Oliver, 1993; Mosqueda, 1993; Trieschmann, 1995; Renwick et al, 1996; Waters and Luker, 1996). Oliver (1993) berates the *'physicality'* of rehabilitation and argues that in many instances the main criterion for success is reduced to whether someone is able to walk. While some contend that this *'preoccupation with physical therapy is slowly being replaced with a more holistic approach'* (Mulley, 1994), progress seems slow.

As Wilkin and Hughes (1986) note, the appeal of an emphasis on function lies in its ability to specify criteria for success and indicate an end point to rehabilitation. The importance of seeing rehabilitation as finite is reflected in the current preoccupation with outcome measurement, which is as prevalent in rehabilitation as in other spheres of health care (Keith and Lipsey, 1993; Guthrie and Harvey, 1994; Cope and Sundance, 1995; Bryant, 1995). Despite quality of life being recognised by many as the primary indicator of successful rehabilitation (Bowling, 1991; 1995; Beckmann and Ditlev, 1992; Renwick et al, 1996), the dominance of functional, and more specifically, physical indicators is apparent when outcome measurement is considered.

Swift (1996) contends that few universal indicators of outcome exist, but a meta-analysis by Evans et al (1995) concludes that they are usually restricted to three broad areas: survival, functional ability and discharge destination. As Higgins (1985) points out, the push to *'close cases'* has always dominated rehabilitation, even in community settings, and from a hospital perspective *'getting the patient home'* is often the ultimate aim (Waters, 1991). With the present onus on economic considerations (Keith, 1995; Dejong and Sutton, 1995; Cope and Sundance, 1995; Landrum et al, 1995), Diller (1990) maintains that a reduction in length of stay will achieve ever greater prominence.

While survival and discharge destination provide clear-cut criteria, the need for further, more elaborate but still quantifiable estimates of outcome, such as functional ability (or other concepts such as quality of life or patient satisfaction) has resulted in considerable store being placed upon scientific measurement in rehabilitation. Tallis (1989) argues that measurement is essential, suggesting that most practitioners are scientifically naïve. Indeed he characterises rehabilitation as *'an ancient art but a scientific infant'* (Tallis, 1992), and is critical of what he terms *'the fallacy of misplaced holism'*, proposing that future rehabilitative efforts should concentrate on reversing impairments rather than reducing disability or handicap. Others see functional scales as lying at the heart of rehabilitation (Studenski and Duncan, 1993), with the production of 'Standardised Functional Assessment Measures' being the ultimate aim (Grainger et al, 1996). Such measures, it is argued, will identify which interventions work and how much input is required (Tallis, 1989), so that specific therapies can be administered at given points in time (Landrum et al, 1995), allowing a predictive relationship to be specified between the *'dose'* of rehabilitation and the *'response'* of the patient (Grainger et al, 1996). Such logic exemplifies the current focus on time-limited, finite and outcome-orientated rehabilitation (Landrum et al, 1995).

Although a physical orientation and measurement model dominates much, although by no means all, of the medical literature, disquiet is expressed by many authors. Some see nothing inherently wrong with measurement *per se* but bemoan the lack of theoretical underpinning in rehabilitation and argue for more than a simple empirical model (Beckmann and Ditlev, 1992; Gleukauf et al, 1993; McFall, 1993; Keith and Lipsey, 1993; Keith, 1995; Renwick and Friefield, 1996). Without adequate critical theorising, constructs tend to become more concrete (McFall, 1993), taking on the mantle of a *'research tradition'* (Porter, 1995), where reality is circumscribed by empirical measurement. Others see this physical domination as reductionist (Bach and Rioux, 1996) and characteristic of a biomedical model with a *'test for every occasion'* (Day and Jankey, 1996). To exacerbate matters, many existing measures not only use physical functioning as a proxy for quality of life (Clark, 1995; Renwick and Friefield, 1996; Brown et al, 1996) but are based on a professional rather than a patient perspective (Bowling, 1991; Renwick and Friefield, 1996). Unfortunately, as will be demonstrated later (see Section 4.1), there is often considerable difference between the way in which professionals and disabled people and their carers perceive the importance of various aspects of their lives.

The above concerns have led many to call for a wider conceptualisation of rehabilitation in which quality of life represents the primary outcome (Anderson and Bury, 1988; Fallowfield, 1990; Bowling, 1991; 1995; Beckmann and Ditlev, 1992; Joseph and Wanlass, 1993; Glueckauf et al, 1993; Renwick et al, 1996; Brown et al, 1996; Renwick and Friefield, 1996; Fitzpatrick, 1996). Furthermore, it is argued that outcome measures should reflect the perspective of the disabled person, rather than professionals (Bowling, 1991; 1995; Day and Jankey, 1996; Schultz and Williamson, 1993; Mechanic, 1995b; Laman and Lankhorst, 1994). This has been summarised by Bowling (1991):

> *'What matters in the 20th Century is how the patient feels, rather than how doctors think they ought to feel on the basis of clinical measurement ... particularly where people are treated for chronic or life threatening conditions, the therapy has to be evaluated in terms of whether it is more or less likely to lead to an outcome of a life worth living in social and psychological, as well as physical terms.'* (p1)

Measures such as the Rehabilitation Activities Profile (Laman and Lankhorst, 1994; Van Bennekom et al, 1995; Lankhorst et al, 1995) reflect attempts to capture more clearly the subjective element of various functional and other parameters. However, substituting concepts such as quality of life for more narrow and limited physical indicators raises other problems. The appeal of functional criteria is that they are relatively easy to measure (Livneh, 1995; Swift, 1996), whereas quality of life is conceptually vague and multifaceted (Fallowfield, 1990; Bowling, 1991; 1995; Brown et al, 1996). If maintaining or enhancing quality of life is seen by some as the *'overriding principle inherent in rehabilitation'* (Brown et al, 1996) its implications are only just beginning to be considered (Renwick et al, 1996). Unfortunately as people *'jump on the bandwagon'* (Brown et al, 1996) quality of life is often treated as synonymous with related concepts such as life satisfaction and morale. Beckmann and Ditlev (1992) contend that many have abandoned attempts to define quality of life as too complex, while others measure it without attempting a definition.

Essentially, as Brown et al (1996) point out, quality of life is a social construct with no inherent meaning outside a social context. Recently there have been attempts to reflect this within measures intended for use in rehabilitation (Felce and Perry, 1996; Renwick and Brown, 1996). For example, Renwick and Brown (1996) define quality of life as *'the degree to which a person enjoys the important possibilities of his/her life'*; achieving this is based on an ongoing interaction between an individual and his or her environment. They suggest three broad domains of measurement, each with sub-areas:

- *being* – reflecting the 'personhood' of an individual on physical, psychological and spiritual levels

- *belonging* – the extent to which as person fits in with their physical, social and community environment

- *becoming* – the degree to which an individual can meet their goals, aspirations and hopes in practical domains, leisure pursuits and opportunities for personal growth.

Measures are being developed in each of the above areas and suggest promise for a more holistic measurement approach to rehabilitation, combining the rigour of measurement with a theoretical model intended to capture the diverse domains of quality of life. This reflects the increasing realisation of the need to develop measures of handicap as well as disability (Harwood et al, 1994).

However, there is also considerable debate about the validity and relevance of outcome measurement of *any* sort. The concept of outcomes suggests a finite input and distinct end-point (Guthrie and Harvey, 1994), allowing the specification of an *'ultimate desirable result'* (Bryant, 1995). This ignores the fact that treatment and support may be lifelong (Keith and Lipsey, 1993); it is now more widely recognised that rehabilitation does not relate just to the acute phase of an illness or disability (Palat, 1992; Dejong and Sutton, 1995) and that goals should be consistent with its phase or stage (Wood, 1993; Keith and Lipsey, 1993; Cope and Sundance, 1995; Brown et al, 1996). This requires that both long-term and short-term goals are set, negotiated and agreed by all parties (Andrews, 1987; Thurgood, 1990; Wood, 1993; Williams, 1994; Guthrie and Harvey, 1994). In these circumstances the notion of an ultimate outcome becomes tenuous at best because goals evolve as progress is made. The addition of such a *temporal* dimension to rehabilitation is important and has implications for the process as a whole and the nurse's role in particular, which will be considered in detail in Chapters 6 and 7.

The emergence of a number of temporal models of illness and disability recognise that physical recovery is only an *'interlude'* in the process of disability (Keith and Lipsey, 1993). Furthermore, it is also now realised that to focus on the disabled person alone is insufficient and that not only the family but the wider community and society as a whole should be included (Blaxter, 1976; Dejong and Sutton; 1995, Price, 1996).

Despite this more holistic orientation critics argue that disability is still mainly seen as a *'personal tragedy'* (Oliver, 1990), thereby locating the problem, and therefore the solution, with the individual rather than with society. Recognition of this is slowly filtering into the rehabilitation literature, with more emphasis on the need to target interventions on the environment (Renwick and Brown, 1996) and society (Ville et al, 1994; Bach and Rioux, 1996; Renwick et al, 1996), whereby rehabilitation acquires social, cultural, religious, moral and ethical implications (Keir, 1996).

Such a conceptualisation extends responsibility for rehabilitation far beyond health professionals and health services, implicating personal social services, leisure, transport and vocational and employment agencies (Beardshaw, 1988). Although such a model has yet fully to penetrate mainstream rehabilitation practice, the fact that it is even being considered owes much to the influence of the International Classification of Impairment, Disability and Handicap (ICIDH) (WHO, 1980).

3.2 The ICIDH: a stimulus for change

There is a general consensus in the literature that publication of the ICIDH stimulated considerable debate about the meaning of, and relationship between, rehabilitation and disablement (Badley et al, 1987; Badley and Lee, 1987; Beardshaw, 1988; Tallis, 1992; Pollock et al, 1993; Keith and Lipsey, 1993; Verbrugge and Jette, 1994; Bowling, 1995; Badley, 1995; Peters, 1995; Brandsma et al, 1995; Dickson, 1996; Renwick and Brown, 1996). The ICIDH is essentially an attempt to *'clarify the consequences of chronic disease by offering a new taxonomy'* (Harwood et al, 1994), to narrow the gap between what health care systems *can do* for people with chronic disease and what they *actually do* (Peters, 1995). This signals *'an important departure from strictly biomedical thinking'* (Peters, 1995) by explicitly including the human consequences of disease. As Peters (1995) points out the ICIDH was not intended to be a definitive solution but to provide a map to help navigate some difficult conceptual terrain. Halbertsma (1995) argues that its main strength is that it includes a social dimension. She contends that the ICIDH has been used widely to obtain diagnostic information, provide the conceptual underpinnings of many health measures, and plan and evaluate therapeutic interventions, particularly in rehabilitation. It has also aided communication within multidisciplinary teams, being used as the basis for a standard terminology in a range of non-medical disciplines.

The classification consists of four primary elements which are represented schematically in the following way (Badley, 1995; Halbertsma, 1995):

Disease $\rightarrow$ Impairment $\rightarrow$ Disability $\rightarrow$ Handicap

where, according to Badley (1995) the arrows $\rightarrow$ signify 'may lead to'. This is seen as an extension of the traditional medical model (Halbertsma, 1995):

Aetiology $\rightarrow$ Pathology $\rightarrow$ Manifestations

While the medical model is useful for preventable or curable disorders it is of limited help in chronic conditions, as it makes no reference to the consequences of a disease, being primarily concerned with causative factors.

Halbertsma (1995) points out the ICIDH, unlike the medical model, is not meant to depict a *causal* relationship but rather that the concepts of impairment, disability and handicap *describe* health problems or health states at a particular time. Thus while there is an element of interdependence between the concepts there is not necessarily a causal relationship. The ICIDH is therefore best seen as an heuristic device. The three elements, for example, often co-exist, describing a differing consequence of the same disease (Harwood et al, 1994; Halbertsma, 1995; Badley, 1995). Badley (1995) suggests that impairments are concerned with the consequences of disease at the level of the body, disability at the level of the person and handicap the social repercussions. Alternatively Halbertsma (1995) characterises these as medical, functional and social/economic perspectives. Although formal definitions of these concepts were provided by the WHO, they are succinctly summarised by Harwood et al (1994):

> '*An* impairment *is any loss or abnormality of physiological or anatomical structure or function (for example shortness of breadth or weakness in a limb). A* disability *is any restriction or lack of ability to perform a task or activity (such as walking, dressing or maintaining continence). A* handicap *is the disadvantage suffered by an individual as a result of ill health due to the inability to fulfil a role which is normal for someone of that age, sex or culture.*' (Harwood et al, 1994 p53 original emphasis)

The ICIDH has stimulated considerable debate, but has also been the subject of criticism. Verbrugge and Jette (1994), for example, identify problems with conceptual clarity, internal consistency and measurement, whereas Dickson (1996) argues that it is often applied incorrectly and medicalises social problems. Although there is some justification to these criticisms, in many ways they are inappropriate. The ICIDH was not intended to specify causal relationships, so the absence of internal consistency is less of an issue, and problems of measurement cannot necessarily be attributed to the theoretical framework from which they are derived. While it is no doubt correct that the ICIDH has been used to medicalise social problems, this is a failure of those who use it rather than of the classification. The ICIDH has been of enormous benefit, stimulating debate and highlighting the personal and social consequences of disease.

One of the ICIDH's positive contributions has been to focus on the experiential consequences of disease – handicap (Grainger, 1986; Harwood et al, 1994; Peters, 1995; Barnitt and Pomeroy, 1995). Paradoxically, this has been the most problematic element (Badley, 1995); for although the ICIDH was intended to move beyond the medical model this has been '*tenacious*' (Beardshaw, 1988). This is partly attributable to the fact that the definition and meaning of handicap poses a number of challenges (Badley, 1995). Consequently, as Peters (1995) argues, although the human experience of disablement provides the '*imperative*' for the ICIDH, the concept of handicap has proved difficult to translate into daily practice, a situation exacerbated in part by the training of most health care professionals and the '*weight of medical history*'.

> '*That biomedical thinking has deeply influenced chronic care and rehabilitation medicine is no surprise, nor is it a surprise that the psychosocial domain of the ICIDH has been the focus of confusion for many trained in the biomedical tradition.*' (Peters, 1995 p137)

In order to overcome this confusion, Peters advocates the inclusion of an '*insider's*' perspective in studies of chronic illness and rehabilitation to counter an outsider's perspective which renders handicap abstract. He called for the application of phenomenological methods and other qualitative approaches, a recognition of the limitations of a linear model and the creation of an explanatory framework in which interaction and interpretation are the keys to understanding. Literature on the experience of chronic illness (reviewed in Chapters 4 and 5) highlights the value of this orientation.

Therefore, Peters suggests that the ICIDH be conceived of as a framework which includes both an outsider's (objective) and insider's (subjective) perspective. He notes that: '*A key issue in successfully addressing disablement, both individually and socially, is understanding where generalisations end and individuality begins*' (Peters, 1995). Essential to this is a better understanding of the meaning of handicap; Badley (1995) provides a useful review of modifications to the ICIDH which have attempted to broaden its scope by including external factors. She points out that the ICIDH is concerned exclusively with the *consequences* of disease, so the influence of external factors, such as the environment, are not included, a major omission which limits the application of the ICIDH. Although Badley (1995) identifies a number of definitions of handicap, these share at least two common elements: all highlight the experiential consequences of a disease and all include some external influences.

Badley (1995) describes several variants of the ICIDH based on this broader interpretation of handicap and suggests that they differ primarily in the role attributed to external factors. Social models of disability view external factors (for example the built environment and societal attitudes) as *causing* disability, evidenced by the failure of society to modify the environment and by the application of the standards of performance of able bodied people as the benchmarks of citizenship. Other models present a more dynamic view in which handicap results from the *interaction* between an individual and the environment. While no single model has, according to Badley (1995), gained overall acceptance, all share the common premise that factors other than impairment and disability are necessary to develop understanding of handicap.

The range of external factors cited seems, *'infinitely large'* (Badley, 1995) and may include, for example, social factors (family, public infrastructure and political and governmental systems) and ecological factors (geography, climate and so on). Verbrugge and Jette (1994) suggested that factors may be extra-individual, such as medical care and rehabilitation, the social and physical environment or intra-individual, such as lifestyle and behaviour or personality. Moreover, external factors may reduce the impact of disability and therefore handicap (for instance, provision of good access to public buildings) or exacerbate such difficulties (for example, Tranter et al (1995) estimate that 25% of public pavements in Wales need urgent repair).

Badley (1995) suggests that there are two broad categories of external factors, those that exist independently of an impairment but become significant when impairment occurs – *'pre-existing factors'* and those that are mobilised as a consequence of impairment, for example technical aids – *'responsive factors'*. Both may exert a moderating or a potentiating effect.

The relationship between external factors, individual perceptions, impairments and the experience of handicap is complex and multifaceted, but an appreciation of it is essential to a full understanding of disablement and is of considerable significance for rehabilitation, indicating that a broad range of variables must be included in assessment and intervention models. Verbrugge and Jette (1994) suggest that disablement is the *'gap between personal capability and environmental demand'* and argue that rehabilitation should either attempt to increase the capability, reduce the demand or both. As Mechanic (1995a) proposes, therefore, barriers in the community are (or should be) a major focus for rehabilitation.

Acknowledging the existence and importance of external barriers is the first step, and these are now more widely accepted; however, there is still the question of whose responsibility it is to address them. This broader view of handicap extends rehabilitation out of the narrow confines of the health service and suggests that action needs to be social, legal and political (Akridge, 1986), but it does not absolve the health services from all responsibility for the social consequences of disease and this, as will be argued later (see Chapter 6), is an area where nurses may play an important role.

3.3 Biopsychosocial and temporal models of disability and rehabilitation

Conceptually related to, but distinct from, the ICIDH are so-called biopsychosocial models of disability and chronic illness. These represent an attempt to broaden the scope of the biomedical model by incorporating a range of other components such as psychological, social, economic, environmental and cognitive factors (James and Minichiello, 1994). A number of such models have been advocated for use in the rehabilitation field (Rolland, 1988; 1994; Shaw and Halliday, 1992; Ward and McIntosh, 1993; Mosqueda, 1993; James and Minichiello, 1994; Pawlson, 1994; Barnitt and Pomeroy, 1995; Talo et al, 1995).

Pawlson (1994) for example called for a *'new paradigm'* of health care which is more relevant to the needs of modern society, and advocates the adoption of a *'chronic complex illness model'* which he contrasts on a number of criteria with the currently prevalent *'acute simple disease model'* (Table 3.1).

Criteria	Acute simple disease model	Chronic complex illness model
Cause	Single agent sufficient	Multiple contributing factors
Basis of disease	Altered physiology (biologic)	Biopsychosocial
Aim of interventions	Normal physiology (cure)	Ameliorate and relieve suffering
Temporal relationship	Single event	Continuous process
Role of patient	Passive recipient	Active participant

Table 3.1: Comparison of chronic complex illness and acute simple disease models
(after Pawlson, 1994)

In terms of rehabilitation, Pawlson (1994) argues that the chronic complex model is more appropriate but that the acute simple approach is usually applied. He suggests that the patient must be the key decision-maker in rehabilitation and sees this as one of the prime indicators of a quality service. Working from a similar premise Robinson (1988) contrasts the *'short-term rehabilitation model'* with the long-term model (Table 3.2). Although not identical to Pawlson's thinking the rationale is consistent.

Short-term rehabilitation model	Long-term rehabilitation model
Focus on impairment/disability	Focus on handicap
Technique orientated	Patient orientated
Doctor as controller	Doctor as co-ordinator
Therapist as agent	Therapist as autonomous
Hospital based	Community based

Table 3.2: The short-term and long-term rehabilitation models
(after Robinson, 1988)

Robinson argues that the long-term model is more appropriate to rehabilitation but that its implementation is hindered by professional rivalry. Interestingly, Robinson (1988) believes that therapists form the ideal bridge linking the two models and the nursing role is hardly considered.

Rather than presenting competing models, as do Pawlson (1994) and Robinson (1988), others outline a more linear, temporal sequence, providing a continuum, which sometimes begins before the onset of disability (or disease/injury) and extends to include handicap. Many such models also suggest the focus of interventions at various stages and indicate which professional group(s) should take a lead role. A comparison of these models, using elements of the ICIDH as an analytic device is presented in Table 3.3.

Model	Level	Stage	Purpose	Responsibility/Focus
Livneh 1995 Tripartite model	Predisease Impairment Disability Handicap	Primary Secondary (crisis) Tertiary (I) ← Tertiary (II) → Tertiary (III)	Reduce/prevent disability Preserve life Minimise disability Compensate for disability Modify environment	Acute medical interventions OT, physio, speech therapist Counselling Social work, vocational Rehabilitation
Hershenson (1990)	Predisease Impairment Disability Handicap	Primary - - - - - Secondary ← Tertiary →	Reduce/prevent disability Reduce functional limitations Prevent limitations becoming handicaps	Public health (environment) Medicine, therapy (person) Rehabilitation counselling (person and environment)
Hunt (1980) (cited by Andrews 1987) The SPREAD model	Predisease Impairment Disability Handicap		**S**pecific control of disease **P**revention of secondary disability **RE**storative measure **AD**aptation	Medical Nursing/therapy Therapy/nursing Therapy/S.W.
Cope and Sundance (1995)	Predisease Impairment Disability Handicap	Physiologic instability Physiologic stability Physiologic maintenance Residential reintegration Community reintegration Productive activity	Preserve life Prevent complications to skin etc. Environment of choice Community of choice Recreation, social activity relevant to life stages and interests	Medicine/intensive nursing Nursing Therapy

Table 3.3: Models of the rehabilitation process

These models are useful in reinforcing the importance of a temporal dimension which extends rehabilitation beyond the acute (crisis) phase, through the restoration of function and minimisation of complications (i.e. disability) to handicap. They are also interesting as they specify where the perceived responsibility for action lies; it is instructive to note that nursing does not appear at all in some and in others it is confined largely to the prevention of complications. This pattern is reflected in much of the general literature on the nurse's role in rehabilitation.

The models summarised in Table 3.3 are based on professional perspectives and reflect, implicitly or explicitly, a number of assumptions. Other temporal and longitudinal models have been described, based on the perceptions of individuals with a chronic illness or disability. These take greater account of the biographical and existential impact of illness and disability and are considered separately, primarily in Section 4.2.

Probably one of the most comprehensive and potentially useful of the professionally derived models, based on a temporal biopsychological disease approach but incorporating a family systems perspective, is described by Rolland (1988; 1994). Rolland argues that this provides a conceptual basis for theory development, research and practice in chronic and life-threatening illness while accounting for the heterogeneity of such conditions. He believes it necessary to account for the diversity and commonality in chronic illness while accommodating qualitative and quantitative variations over time which, he contends, requires a move away from biological classifications to incorporate psychosocial aspects. He outlines the *'therapeutic quadrangle model'* which incorporates the perspectives of the disabled or ill person, the carer/ family, the professionals involved and the nature of the disease or impairment.

It is interesting to compare the characteristics of Rolland's model with Morse and Johnson's (1991) criteria of adequacy for any framework claiming to account for the complexity of chronic illness. They advocate that any model must:

- consider the entire duration of the illness

- be responsive to its dynamic and changing nature

- reflect or incorporate a patient's perspective

- consider similarities across illness experiences

- account for the context of illness, including the experience of significant others.

The congruence between these criteria and the way that Rolland characterises his model is impressive, especially when it is considered that, as far as can be established, the criteria and the model were constructed without reference to each other.

As will become apparent in Sections 4.2 and 7.2, accommodating many experiential elements of chronic illness as described by individuals themselves further adds to the potential usefulness of approaches such as Rolland's. Moreover, Rolland incorporates a family systems perspective which recognises the essential contribution of family members to the rehabilitation process. Family systems approaches have recently become far more prominent in the nursing literature, as witnessed by the emergence of a journal dedicated to this aspect of practice (the *Journal of Family Nursing*).

Rolland (1988; 1994) presents an overarching model, developed primarily from clinical experience and a synthesis of the literature rather than research-based empirical work. Despite the appeal of such models there is still a need to consider the relevance of several theoretical perspectives. Prior to turning attention to a number of theories and concepts derived from the literature, the next chapter identifies a number of recurring themes, beginning with patient involvement.

4.1 Patient involvement and empowerment

The need to incorporate multiple perspectives within the rehabilitation process figures prominently in the literature (Bowles et al, 1995; Kleinmann, 1995; Pollock et al, 1993; Evans et al, 1995; Sheppard, 1994a; 1994b) with particular emphasis on the involvement of disabled people themselves (Keane et al, 1987; Becker and Kaufman, 1988; Waters, 1987; 1991; Joseph and Wanlass, 1993; Robinson et al, 1993; Howell, 1994; Pawlson, 1994; Preston, 1994; Sheppard, 1994a; 1994b; Scullion, 1995; Mechanic, 1995b; 1995b; Van Bennekom et al, 1995; Price, 1996). Great store is placed on active participation in treatment and decision-making (Nordstrom, 1980), with many considering that disabled people should take a lead in goal-setting (Jackson, 1987; Sheppard, 1994a; 1994b; Guthrie and Harvey, 1994; Bowles et al, 1995) by establishing a *'therapeutic narrative'* (Kleinmann, 1995) and forging a partnership with those delivering care (Renwick et al, 1996).

Patient-centred care has been advocated for some time (Evers, 1981) and more recently notions of empowerment (Beardshaw, 1988) have become more prevalent, resulting in initiatives such as the *Patient's Charter*. Indeed Fulford (1996) considers that few now stop to question what patient-centred care actually means. Its rise to prominence is partly a consequence of the application of consumerist principles to health care in general (Williamson, 1992) and rehabilitation in particular (Dejong and Sutton, 1995; Landrum et al, 1995). However, this offers only a partial and not particularly convincing account. A more significant influence is the realisation that a full appreciation of rehabilitation and the effects of chronic illness and disability can only be gained if the subjective views of disabled people are taken into account (Radley and Green, 1987; Morse and Johnson, 1991; Corbin and Strauss, 1991; Baker and Stern, 1993; Thorne, 1993; Jensen and Allen, 1994; Radley, 1994; Luborsky, 1995; Fife, 1995; Peplau, 1995). Since they have expert knowledge of their own condition (Strauss et al, 1984; Robinson, 1988; Beardshaw, 1988; Corbin and Strauss, 1991; Thorne, 1993; Lamb and Stempel, 1994; Donnelly, 1995; Marris, 1996) they can also provide vital insights into the appropriateness and acceptability of interventions.

The creation of a genuine partnership between professionals and disabled people does not come easily, however, requiring good channels of communication and mutual trust and respect. Initially, especially following acute illness or injury, it may be more appropriate for professionals to take the lead (Sheppard, 1994a; 1994b; Jelles et al, 1995), as patients may lack the knowledge to make meaningful decisions or be too ill or frail to participate actively (Jelles et al, 1995). Subsequently professionals may need to teach disabled people to take greater control (Jelles et al, 1995) or alter their perceptions that professionals should be *'doing'* things for them (Sheppard, 1994a; 1994b). Establishing the trust necessary to achieve this requires effort from both parties (Jackson, 1987; Strauss et al, 1984; Thorne, 1993; Moss-Morris and Petrie, 1994), as there may be considerable differences in perception between professionals and disabled people on important parameters (Strauss et al, 1984; Higgins, 1985; Robinson, 1988; Beardshaw, 1988; Anderton et al, 1989; Schüssler, 1992; Worthington, 1994; Porter, 1995; Clark, 1995; NOP, 1996), particularly when professionals rely heavily on objective criteria.

Such criteria are of limited use as there is often little congruence between an individual's objective circumstances and subjective perceptions of their situation (Blaxter, 1976; Robinson, 1988; Ben-Sira, 1989; Pollock, 1993; Dangoor and Florian, 1994; Peters, 1995; Fitzpatrick, 1996). Such differences in perception may be so great that, according to Peters (1995), clinicians and disabled people might as well be occupying *'different universes'*, and in these circumstances patients often see their prescribed treatment as irrelevant (Wood, 1993).

Numerous studies and personal accounts confirm the difficulties experienced by disabled people in interactions with health care professionals. Compounding such difficulties, Peters (1995) argues that professionals often see disabled people's perceptions as wrong, implicitly discounting the value of their experience. This is not an isolated conclusion; the expertise and knowledge held by disabled people is often ignored or overlooked, particularly during periods of hospitalisation (Strauss et al, 1984; Beardshaw, 1988; Corbin and Strauss, 1991; Marris, 1996). The limited involvement that does occur is often tokenistic (Beardshaw, 1988) and disquiet over the quality of communication between professionals, particularly doctors, and disabled people has been noted for some time (Blaxter, 1976).

Unfortunately, those who voice concerns are frequently seen as *'bolshy'* (Robinson, 1988) and disabled people are often *'astonished and horrified'* at their treatment by professionals (Thorne, 1993), who can be *'uncomprehending or downright hostile'* (Marris, 1996). Oliver (1986; 1990; 1993) considers this a reflection of the power differentials inherent in health care, a point reiterated by Marris (1996) who suggests that disabled people, who often have the least power, usually experience the worst the NHS has to offer. Although initiatives such as the *Patient's Charter* may have addressed this situation, recent surveys of disabled people suggest there is scope for considerable improvement (NOP, 1996; Baker et al, 1997).

Waters (Waters, 1991; Waters and Luker, 1996) notes the largely passive role accorded to patients receiving rehabilitation in hospital, exemplified by the use of rehabilitation as a verb – something that staff do to patients.

It seems, therefore, that despite the rhetoric of involvement and empowerment, such ideals are rarely realised. If progress is to be made, professionals must gain a wider appreciation of the impact of chronic illness and disability from the perspectives of affected individuals. Fortunately a wealth of literature provides insights into these.

4.2 Incorporating the perspectives of the disabled person

Guthrie and Harvey (1994) argue that rehabilitation *'belongs'* to the person with disability and as such their goals are of central importance. Although this does not mean the disabled person should be left to make decisions in isolation nor that their view necessarily always prevails (Fulford, 1996) there should, as a minimum, be agreement about the goals of care between the disabled person (and family) and the professionals involved (Nordstrom, 1980; Robinson, 1988; Becker and Kaufmann, 1988; Ward and McIntosh, 1993; McDaniel and Bach, 1994; Sheppard, 1994a; 1994b) with one of the key tasks being to assist those needing rehabilitation to set realistic goals (Ireys et al, 1994; Metcalfe, 1995; Knight, 1996). As illustrated previously, however, this is rarely the case, with a professional hegemony still being apparent (Strauss and Corbin, 1988; Oliver, 1993).

If the experience of handicap is to be rendered *'real'* (Peters, 1995) and meaningful interventions designed, professionals must understand how people make sense of their illness and disability (Robinson, 1988; Miller, 1992a; Baker and Stern, 1993; Price, 1996). This involves considering such questions as *'what is it like to be ill?'* (Morse and Johnson, 1991) and *'what is it like to live with illness in a world of health?'* (Radley, 1994). Addressing these questions is essential to harmonise understandings and perspectives on disability (Luborsky, 1995). For example Forsythe (1988), a doctor, describes how her usual detached medical approach proved inadequate when confronted with diagnosis of her illness; only when she appreciated that the disease (multiple sclerosis) could not be separated from herself could she begin to make sense of her situation.

The ability to create and sustain individually salient meanings about illness and disability appears to lie at the heart of successful adaptation and coping (Lazarus, 1993; Jensen and Allen, 1994; Fife, 1995; Klienmann, 1995). This often involves continuous reconstruction, especially if the illness runs a changing course (Corbin and Strauss, 1988; Thompson, 1992; Rolland, 1988; 1994). If people with chronic illness and disability are to construct serviceable meanings, however, they need to trust their own experience and have this validated by others. As Charmaz (1983) suggests, it is the paradox of chronic illness to place increasing reliance on others for self-validation at a time when relationships are more likely to be strained and problematic. The perceptions of professionals are often particularly important in validating the experience of people with illness and disability (Charmaz, 1983; 1987; Howell, 1994; Carson, 1995), yet the importance of such validation is seldom explicitly recognised by professionals involved in rehabilitation.

From the literature on the individual experience of chronic illness or disability, three core clusters of ideas emerge and underpin a number of the models which have been developed. Although these concepts are distinct there is a degree of overlap, suggesting an interactive and dynamic relationship between the *existential, biographical* and *temporal* dimensions of illness and disability.

Loss of a sense of 'self' has long been recognised as one of the most devastating effects of illness and disability (Blaxter, 1976; Bury, 1982; Charmaz, 1983; 1987; Corbin and Strauss, 1988; 1991; 1992; Robinson, 1988; Beckmann and Ditlev, 1992; Carricaburu and Pierret, 1995); indeed Robinson (1988) suggests it often results in a *'demolished identity'*. Reconstructing a new and equally valued sense of self is a key task in adapting to chronic illness (Charmaz, 1983; 1987; Robinson, 1988), for as Beckmann and Ditlev (1992) contend a new sense of 'I' must be created before recovery and adaptation can begin in earnest. Kleinmann (1995) argues that this means accommodating to an existential world comprising conflicting feelings of hope, transcendence and despair.

In other words, living with chronic illness is about *'being'* rather than *'doing'* (Robinson, 1988), yet the prime focus of rehabilitation remains on doing. Indeed it is often difficult to find an acknowledgement of the importance of existential factors in the mainstream rehabilitation literature, and the *'judgement, wisdom and ingenuity'* that professionals should bring to bear (Strauss et al, 1984) is seldom apparent. Barnard (1995) notes that professionals thrive on *'dramatic results'* and feel a failure when these prove elusive. He advocates developing the skills of *'empathetic witnessing'* to help ill and disabled people make sense of the *'existential paradox'* they experience, caught between increased awareness of their mortality and the need to transcend their illness.

Others also speak of transcending illness and restoring a sense of living a valuable life (Gerhardt, 1990; Milz, 1992; Marris, 1996), as only in this way will disabled people achieve a sense of health and wellness (Howell, 1994; Jensen and Allen, 1994) and be able to live life as a *'healthy ill person'* (Milz, 1992). Synthesising the results of 112 qualitative studies on wellness-illness, Jensen and Allen (1994) describe a new theory of wellness in which healthy people may not necessarily experience wellness if their life is not *'integrated'* while, conversely, individuals with disease may feel well if they integrate and accommodate the disease into their lives. It is recognised that rehabilitation has paid too much attention to illness and disability at the expense of health and wellbeing (RCN, 1994). It is suggested that if the balance is to be redressed, the existential components of the illness experience must be taken into account.

Two complementary concepts, also necessary for more complete understanding of illness and disability are *biography* and *temporality*. Reconstructing a sense of 'I' (Bury, 1982; Beckmann and Ditlev, 1992) is impossible without reference to the past and to a number of potential futures (Gerhardt, 1990), and it is often necessary to reconceptualise the past in order to construct a meaningful future (Jensen and Allen, 1994; Fife, 1995; Luborsky, 1995; Klienmann, 1995). One of the most significant effects of chronic illness and disability is that it separates the past from the present and the present from the future, rendering biography *'discontinuous'* (Corbin and Strauss, 1988). Restoring continuity necessitates a fundamental rethinking of biography and self-concept (Bury, 1982), with biography in this context serving to unite the existential and temporal dimensions of illness and disability.

A number of authors explore the complex interactions between these subjective experiences and propose models which potentially provide a better understanding of how people live with illness and disability (Charmaz, 1987; Corbin and Strauss, 1988; 1991; 1992; Morse and Johnson, 1991; Thorne, 1993; Radley, 1994). While they all offer valuable insights which may help to extend and improve current rehabilitation practice, the models of Corbin and Strauss, Morse and Johnson and Thorne are most widely cited in the nursing literature, and are therefore explored further below.

Based on 30 years of research in chronic illness and disability Corbin and Strauss (1988; 1991; 1992) present a *'trajectory model'* which reflects the existential, temporal and biographical components noted above. The key concept, that of a 'trajectory', relates not only the physiological unfolding of an illness but incorporates the diverse range of experiences involved. Central to the model is the idea that this trajectory can be shaped or managed, but that achieving this requires three broad categories of 'work':

- *illness-related work*: managing the disease and its treatment

- *biographical work*: to reconstitute identity and recast biography

- *everyday work*: occupation, marriage, child rearing and so on.

The relative emphasis placed on these types of work varies as the trajectory of the illness unfolds, and is influenced by the phase, described as: *initial crisis and diagnosis, comeback, stable, unstable and downward*. Corbin and Strauss argue that rehabilitation is often confined to the comeback phase but that the disabled or ill person and family require help in all phases. They believe that disabled people and their families develop a trajectory plan and that professionals must understand this factor.

Corbin and Strauss' model has a number of implications for practice as it highlights the long-term nature of chronic illness and the need to account for the illness phase and the trajectory scheme if professionals are to support the 'work' of disabled people and their families. Although the model has been criticised for not including a nursing perspective (Baines and Oglesby, 1991), the trajectory framework, as demonstrated in Section 8.2, has been developed and applied in nursing-related contexts.

Morse and Johnson (1991) developed the *'illness constellation model'*, which they argue is more comprehensive than alternatives such as the medical model or a stress-coping approach. The model comprises four stages:

- *uncertainty*, in which the individual and family suspect or detect signs of illness and attempt to interpret them

- *disruption* begins when it is appreciated that the illness is real and help is sought; there is now more active involvement of significant others and a growing reliance on the health care system

- *striving to regain self*, in which there is an attempt to make sense of the illness, renegotiate roles and set goals

- *regaining wellness* is concerned with achieving mastery and a sense of control.

Morse and Johnson (1991) described a number of sub-processes in each of stage of the model, and outline the actions taken by both the ill person and their family. The key variable underpinning the entire process is *'minimising suffering'* which:

> *'... consists of a variety of strategies directed at reducing the physical and psychological discomfort of illness, the social distress extending from changed roles and responsibilities and the uncertainty of the unknown future.'* (p338)

Morse and Johnson (1991) recognise the need for further empirical and conceptual work to elaborate upon the dimensions of suffering, but suggest that their model provides a more holistic approach, as it is based on studies of human experience which incorporate the perspectives of the ill person and significant others. In developing their approach further they consider:

> *'In particular, the role of the family needs to remain at the forefront of illness research. Too often the illness experience has been conceptualised as individualistic rather than reciprocal ... family and friends are intimately involved in and affected by the life of the ill individual and the impact that illness has on these individuals needs to be included.'* (p359)

The importance of family carers will be considered in more detail in Section 4.3.

In a later paper Morse collaborates with O'Brien to present another temporal model which describes the transition from victim to patient to disabled person (Morse and O'Brien, 1995). This was also developed using a grounded theory methodology, specifically with individuals who had suffered serious traumatic injury. As with all the temporal models it comprises a number of discrete but overlapping stages:

- *Vigilance*: becoming engulfed; this begins with a need (in conscious patients) to stay alive and ends when care is relinquished to competent (professional) caregivers.

- *Disruption*: involves taking time out; there are periods of disorientation and a changed perception of the world which ends when the reality of the trauma is recognised and the struggle to accommodate it begins.

- *Enduring the self*: confronting and regrowing; individuals learn to endure the results of their trauma and start the work of healing.

- *Striving to regain self*: this constitutes the 'real' work of rehabilitation in which there are efforts to know and trust the altered body and accept the consequences.

The basic process underpinning the model is that of *'preserving self'*, which involves the use of various strategies as the illness experience unfolds. The final stage of rehabilitation requires the individual to acknowledge his or her disability and create an acceptable sense of self. This is essential to successful rehabilitation and the authors argue that nurses must appreciate *'the enormity of the experience of the patient'* before they can help the person to adapt. As already noted, however, health care professionals often fail to consider fully the patient's experience. This lies at the heart of the model outlined by Thorne (1993).

Thorne (1993) like others (Strauss et al, 1984; Strauss and Corbin, 1988) places considerable emphasis on the experiences of disabled people within the health care system. She argues that acute and chronic illnesses differ radically in their genesis and impact. Consequently the needs of individuals with chronic illness are poorly catered for in a system geared mainly towards the *'miracle cure'*. If things are to improve, there has to be a recognition of chronic illness *'as a complex social phenomenon emerging from factors inherent in a disease, in a society and in a health care system'*. Thorne describes the experiences of chronically ill people in the health care system as ranging from *'frustrating and exhausting to the horrifying, demanding and dehumanising'*. This leaves most people feeling critical and distrustful.

In negotiating their relationship with health care providers, Thorne (1993) describes how chronically ill people begin by feeling *'naïve trust'* which turns to disenchantment and eventually, for many, to a *'guarded alliance'*. Here patients recognise that *they* are the experts and come to realise that there is little that health care professionals can do for them. She also describes a number of consequent relationships typically developed between disabled people and health professionals:

- *hero worship* where reliance is placed on one particular health professional who is both knowledgeable and sensitive

- *resignation* giving up and taking a largely passive role

- *consumerism* treating the health care system as any other 'product'

- *team player* the 'ideal' scenario is a blend of hero worship and consumerism in which mutual trust develops between the disabled person and the professionals involved. However, this rarely occurs due to the failure of professionals to recognise the expertise of the disabled person.

Consistent with other models (Corbin and Strauss, 1988; 1991; 1992) Thorne (1993) uses the metaphor of *'work'* to describe the active role that disabled people play and argues that there are various types of work depending on the stage of acuity or chronicity, including health maintenance, emotional work, managing acute episodes and dealing with hospitalisation. This is consistent with the notion of an *'illness career'* (Price, 1996), which represents another manifestation of the temporal nature of chronic illness.

This section has presented a necessarily condensed overview of a number of models of the experience of illness and disability developed from the accounts of ill and disabled people themselves. However, a number of key themes have emerged which are important to improving rehabilitation practice. These reflect the need to incorporate individuals' subjective experience and the existential, biographical and temporal dimensions of illness. Central to many of the frameworks is the active involvement of family carers and relatives, which is discussed below.

4.3   The involvement of family carers

As with disabled people the literature is unequivocal about the need for family carers to be active participants in rehabilitation (Beardshaw, 1988; Strauss et al, 1984; Morse and Johnson, 1991; Joseph and Wanlass, 1993; Eubanks, 1990; James and Minichiello, 1994; Williams, 1994; Woods and Lewis, 1995; Martin, 1995; Lyons et al, 1995; Guthrie and Harvey, 1994; Cope and Sundance, 1995; Donnelly, 1995; Philp, 1996). It has been asserted that family carers represent the *'key to rehabilitation'* (Weeks and O'Connor, 1994) and that their importance *'can't be exaggerated'* (Twinning, 1996). It is suggested that their needs for education, skills and support must be assessed prior to discharge (Cope and Sundance, 1995), especially when they may be at risk of ill health themselves (Schultz and Williamson, 1993; Brummel-Smith, 1993). This is particularly relevant with the present emphasis on community care.

The importance of family carers in making a reality of community care is beyond doubt (Nolan et al, 1996); they provide far more than physical tending. The presence of a supportive family carer, particularly a spouse or partner, is often essential to maintaining morale and positive adaptation in disabled people (Robinson, 1988; Thompson and Pitts, 1992; Woods and Lewis, 1995; Lyons et al, 1995; Marris, 1996), but policy to support family carers has, until the introduction of the Carers (Recognition and Services) Act (1995) been largely implicit and poorly developed (Twigg and Atkin, 1994; Nolan et al, 1996). Consequently the rationale for supporting carers is inadequately conceptualised, and services generally fail to respond to their changing needs (Nolan et al, 1996). This is particularly noticeable at key transition points, for example, when carers take on their role for the first time or relinquish their role when the cared-for person enters residential care. The *'taking it on'* stage of caregiving (Nolan et al, 1996) is particularly relevant in the context of rehabilitation.

Little attention has been given to the way carers *'take on'* their role (Given and Given, 1991; Nolan and Grant, 1992a; Stewart et al, 1993), but studies suggest that they usually do so without having exercised a genuine choice (Taraborrelli, 1993), and are often unaware of the extent and nature of their responsibilities (Allen et al, 1983; Lewis and Meredith, 1988a; 1988b; Bell and Gibbons, 1989; Nolan and Grant, 1992b). There is little professional input at this time and carers are rarely fully prepared, physically or psychologically, for their role, frequently lacking the necessary knowledge and skills (Braithwaite, 1990; Stewart et al, 1993; Harvath et al, 1994; Kemp, 1993; Lea, 1994). Carers acquire knowledge and skills largely by trial and error, which has been described as *'flailing about'* (Stewart et al, 1993). They have a particular need for information which is often unmet (Thorne, 1993) and according to Strauss et al (1984) they are at the *'bottom of the institutional hierarchy of information'*. If carers' needs are assessed at all they are often *'tacked on'* at the end of the rehabilitation process (Bowles et al, 1995) reinforcing Waters and Luker's (1996) suggestion that carers do not figure until the point of discharge.

Taking on the caregiving role can be a major stressor, involving a number of tasks: emotional, physical, relational; and a range of emotions: guilt, anger, resentment (Thompson and Pitts, 1992), but how carers are prepared for this is rarely addressed and little attention is given to the knowledge and skills they require or the resources they may possess (Kemp, 1993). The emergence of family system models and their application in a rehabilitative context (Doherty and Campbell, 1988; Knafl and Deatrick, 1990; Biegel et al, 1991; Shaw and Halliday, 1992; Stetz et al, 1994; Curry, 1995) has provided new impetus and direction but there is still a need for a temporal model of the caregiving experience which indicates how carers' needs may change over time. Nolan et al (1996) have recently presented such a model; following a review of a number of earlier models, they outline a six-stage sequence:

- building on the past
- recognising the need
- taking it on
- working through it
- reaching the end
- a new beginning.

Nolan et al (1996) argue that caregiving has both common elements and unique components and that these must be taken into account when planning interventions so that support is relevant to the appropriate stage. In order to operationalise this approach they suggest a basis for assessment and intervention with family carers, the *'carers as experts'* model, which they argue helps to focus explicit attention to carers' needs. This is important, as most interventions with carers are poorly planned, *ad hoc* and often lack an explicit rationale (Twigg and Atkin, 1994; Nolan et al, 1994).

The *'carers as experts'* approach potentially provides a more elegant and appropriate model to frame professional interactions with carers. Caring is seen as comprising a number of interrelated practical, cognitive, emotional and relational components in which it is necessary for the carer to become skilled to provide effective care. The level and type of skill required will vary according to the stage of the caregiving history and the demands faced by the carer.

The model is based on the premise that as carers progress through their caring history they gain varying degrees of expertise, much along the lines described by Benner (1984) and Eraut (1994), as relating to professional expertise. Utilising data from several studies Nolan et al (1996) suggest that family carers go through an almost identical process, albeit starting from a different vantage point. Professional expertise usually begins with formal training in which the rules and basic competencies are introduced. However, only when these are practised and refined can genuine expertise begin to develop. Family carers on the other hand usually do not have the luxury of formal training and are lucky to get even basic information or advice when taking on their role (Nolan and Grant, 1992b). Consequently their skills develop largely by trial and error (Stewart et al, 1993; Harvath et al, 1994), potentially prolonging the route to expertise. The primary goal of the *'carers as experts'* model is to work with carers and help them to recognise deficits in their knowledge and skills so that these can be developed. The level of support needed will depend significantly on the stage of the caregiving history. For new carers just about to take on the caring role (Nolan et al, 1994) it is important to ensure they are able to make an informed choice and are willing and able to provide the required care.

A key concept here is that of *'preparedness'* (Archbold et al, 1992) – the extent to which carers feel competent to take on their role. High levels of preparedness, in terms of the necessary knowledge, skills and emotional support, are associated with lower levels of depression (Archbold et al, 1992; Harvath et al, 1994). Where carers feel ill-prepared for their role and are faced with an unpredictable situation, levels of burden are higher (Braithwaite, 1990). Taraborrelli (1993) argues that most carers *'take it on'* in a state of *'initial innocence'* in which they have little information and advice and are generally ignorant of both the extent and the nature of the care they will be expected to deliver. This is by no means an uncommon finding (Allen et al, 1983; Lewis and Meredith, 1988a; 1988b; Bell and Gibbons, 1989; Pitkeathley, 1990; Nolan and Grant, 1992a). Moreover, there appears to be little professional input at this time, and the limited support that is offered is usually confined to the physical aspects of care (Stewart et al, 1993). These considerations are important in the context of rehabilitation; with the trend towards ever more rapid hospital discharge set to continue (Wistow, 1995) there is often little time in hospital devoted to assisting new carers develop their knowledge and skills. Far more attention needs to be paid to how carers can be supported and nurses have a potentially key role in this process.

On the other hand, when assessments are conducted with carers who have been in their role for some time, it must be recognised that they are likely to have developed their own expertise (Nolan and Grant, 1992a). If this is the case, assessors must adopt a strategy that recognises carers' unique knowledge and seeks to blend it creatively with their own professional expertise. It is here that the balance between what Harvath et al (1994) term *local knowledge* and *cosmopolitan knowledge* is important.

These authors argue that carers have local knowledge – expertise of their unique situation – particularly the way the cared-for person responds to his or her illness. It has been suggested that carers have three primary types of local knowledge: knowledge of the cared-for person's illness or disability; knowledge of the cared-for person's normal behaviour and biographical knowledge of past and present interests, likes, hopes and aspirations (Nolan and Grant, 1992a). Cosmopolitan knowledge, on the other hand, is more global. It is not concerned with the specifics of a situation but the generalities. Harvath et al (1994) suggest that the skilful use of these differing types of knowledge will result in the most profitable interactions between carers and service providers.

Nurses usually have the closest contact with families and are in the best position to develop the sort of intimate knowledge of family circumstances needed to blend knowledge most successfully. To achieve this, however, will mean a reorientation of the nurse's role to that of facilitator and enabler rather than doer or provider, giving greater recognition to the emotional demands faced by carers. As Brody (1995) notes, there is a marked tendency for services to focus on elements of care that are tangible and easy to describe and to neglect the emotional elements such as conflict, guilt, anxiety and depression because they are *too slippery*. However, not until such 'slippery' elements are addressed will policy and practice begin to respond adequately to the needs of many carers. This does not mean that practical help should be neglected but rather that carers require a range of interventions tailored to their own circumstances.

On the basis of the literature it is apparent that despite considerable rhetoric about empowering and involving both disabled people and their carers in the rehabilitation process, this is rarely achieved in any meaningful way. Although the reasons are complex, they hinge largely on professionals' reliance on objective factors compounded by their failure fully to acknowledge the importance of subjective perceptions and the tendency to ignore or override sources of knowledge other than their own. As the literature on team-working attests, such disparate perspectives are not confined to professionals and disabled people and their carers, but are also manifest between differing groups of professionals. This leads to a consideration of another prominent theme in the rehabilitation literature: team-working.

4.4   Team-working: fulfilling the reborn certainty

One of the most pervasive concepts within the literature on rehabilitation is team-working. This is often seen as being central to rehabilitation practice despite the fact that there is little evidence for its effectiveness (Walley, 1986; Thurgood, 1990; Henderson et al, 1990; Waters, 1991; Keith, 1991; Preston, 1994; Walker, 1995; Waters and Luker, 1996). Keith (1991) traces the history of team-working in rehabilitation and suggests that although it was little used before World War II, from the 1950s to the 1970s it was unchallenged as the best way to organise and deliver care. However, as with a number of concepts pertaining to rehabilitation, it remains ill-defined and its supposed benefits are largely an act of faith.

Over 20 years ago Halstead (1976) reviewed the literature on 25 years of team-working and concluded that the concept had become a *'catch phrase'* and a *'platitude almost without meaning'*. He found that most of the literature in support of teamwork was opinion, much of the rest offered a simple description of team-working based on personal experience and anecdote with only a *'tiny proportion'* providing evidence of its putative advantages. Others have since reached similar conclusions (Øvretveit, 1990; Keith, 1991; McGrath, 1991; Wood, 1993; Evans et al, 1995; Waters and Luker, 1996; Mumma and Nelson, 1996).

Following the explosion of knowledge in health care, the increasing complexity of treatment regimens and the rise in specialisation (Rothberg, 1981; Wood, 1993) team-working was seen to represent a compromise between the benefits of specialisation and the need for continuity of care (Rothberg, 1981). It has now become universally accepted but remains poorly defined (Rothberg, 1981; McGrath, 1991). The original emphasis was on the multidisciplinary team, with each member contributing their skills and expertise but remaining distinct from other disciplines. Over the last 15 years, however, more reliance has been placed on the interdisciplinary team which is seen to provide a synergy lacking in multidisciplinary models (Rothberg, 1981; Halstead et al, 1986). Initially achieving prominence in the US, the principles of interdisciplinary practice have gained acceptance in the UK and are enthusiastically advocated (RCN, 1994; Fulford, 1996), being seen to offer a *'balance of evaluative considerations'* (Fulford, 1996). Moreover in contrast to the multidisciplinary team which is *'discipline orientated'*, the interdisciplinary team is more in step with the present consumerist ethos as it is considered to be *'patient-orientated'* (Jelles et al, 1995). Diller (1990) suggests that the interdisciplinary team, like a supermarket, provides all that is required in one place.

However, despite unbridled enthusiasm for team-working in numerous government reports and policy statements, there is little evidence for its effectiveness. It also has potential problems and unless carefully orchestrated may prove *'a recipe for disaster'* (Wood, 1993), bringing out the worst in people (Øvretveit, 1993). McGrath (1991), synthesising a number of disparate definitions of teamwork, identifies three elements necessary for effective teamwork:

- a shared and explicit set of aims

- members recognising and valuing different roles

- structures to facilitate smooth working.

Certainly a consensus on aims and objectives is widely regarded as essential (Fairhurst, 1981; Wood, 1993; Schut and Stam, 1994; Hastings, 1996), as are clear channels of communication and a commitment to the team's goals (Thurgood, 1990; Rothberg, 1981; Wood, 1993; Schut and Stam, 1994; Øvretveit, 1993; Halstead et al, 1986; Jelles et al, 1995; Hastings, 1996).

Successful team-working also requires an investment of time and a dedicated infrastructure including team-orientated meetings (Halstead et al, 1986) and case conferences (Rothberg, 1981; Jelles et al, 1995), together with procedures to recognise and deal with potential conflict (Rothberg, 1981; Øvretveit, 1993). It is generally acknowledged that no single team member can claim leadership as of right (Rothberg, 1981; Thurgood, 1990), although this role is often assumed by the senior medical member (RCP, 1986) despite the fact that they are frequently not the most actively involved person (Wood, 1993).

Paradoxically the very requirements of successful team-working appear to be the most difficult to achieve, a situation exacerbated in rehabilitation due to the numerous disciplines involved (Fairhurst, 1981; Beardshaw, 1988) and the fact that rehabilitation practice crosses agency as well as professional divides (Larsson, 1995; Hastings, 1996).

Underscoring the difficulties faced by team-working are deep-rooted traditions of practice and belief often based on different professional values and theoretical orientations (Beardshaw, 1988; Keith, 1991; Waters, 1991; Milz, 1992). Unfortunately such differences, values and beliefs are often implicit rather than explicit (Qualls and Czirr, 1988) and emanate from the *'assumptive worlds'* of practitioner groups or the local *'culture of the office'* (Twigg and Atkin, 1994), making them all the more difficult to address. Consequently differing groups may speak varying professional languages (Jelles et al, 1995) with multiple realities and interpretations of team roles often existing (Fairhurst, 1981). Issues of potential role overlap are rarely acknowledged and addressed (Waters, 1991; Waters and Luker, 1996) and many of the difficulties teams experience emanate from a failure to understand and value the contribution of other members (Qualls and Czirr, 1988; McGrath, 1991; Barnitt and Pomeroy, 1995). Considerable status problems can ensue (Mullins, 1989; Wood, 1993; Neal, 1995), resulting in jealousy and a lack of co-operation (Benson and Ducanies, 1995) and even sabotage and manipulation (Mullins, 1989). Although such difficulties are often attributed to personality clashes (Wood, 1993), Øvretveit (1993) believes they can be overcome through good organisation, clear channels of communication and robust support mechanisms.

It seems that the organisational infrastructure within which most teams operate militate against their chances of success. Staff turnover does little to promote stability (Halstead et al, 1986; Beardshaw, 1988; Sheppard, 1994a; 1994b) and the shift system worked by core members makes regular attendance at meetings problematic (Sheppard, 1994a; 1994b). Wood (1993) also considers that the existence of separate management hierarchies, most manifest in nursing, does little to resolve potential leadership difficulties and conflicts of loyalty.

If the situation is stark within teams of different disciplines, difficulties are compounded when cross-agency working is considered. The promotion of cross-agency working has underpinned UK health and social services policy for some 30 years (Hunter and Wistow, 1991), as recently promulgated in such euphemisms as a *'seamless service'* (Nolan, 1992). However, Beardshaw (1988) contends that agencies have not started to ask basic questions let alone answer them. Simply exhorting agencies to work together is insufficient (Henwood, 1992), particularly when their *raison d'être* reflects differing cultures and value systems (Rowbottom, 1992).

The ultimate conundrum is perhaps reflected in the principle of patient and carer involvement. As previously highlighted it is now generally considered essential that patients and disabled people and their family carers must play a full and active role in rehabilitation. Logically therefore they are key members of the interdisciplinary team, (Evers, 1981; Fairhurst, 1981; McGrath, 1991), but this is rarely the case and the lack of even professional consensus on team function and purpose suggests that genuine involvement of disabled people and their carers is likely to remain little other than an ideal to which to aspire, as Rothberg (1981) characterised the interdisciplinary team.

McCoy (1983) coined the term *'reborn certainty'* to capture the tendency for services to be perceived as successful simply by a periodic restatement of their worth rather than any evidence of their usefulness. The same might well be said of teamwork.

4.5   Rehabilitation: neglected areas in the literature

Although the literature on rehabilitation is extensive, some potentially important areas have received relatively little attention, including differences by race, culture, gender and class and the location of rehabilitative activity.

A number of authors have highlighted the importance of the influence of race, ethnicity and culture to the way that individuals or groups interpret and respond to illness, particularly chronic illness (Anderton et al, 1989; Masterson, 1994; Young, 1995; Luborsky, 1995; George and Young, 1996). However, such factors receive scant attention both in the rehabilitation literature and in practice (Masterson, 1994; George and Young, 1996), despite the fact that differing ethnic and cultural beliefs may not be consistent with many principles underpinning rehabilitation practice in western society. For example, Anderton et al (1989) argue that the concept of normalisation, which has shaped much of the rehabilitation agenda, may be irrelevant to the way certain cultures construct chronic illness. Similarly Luborsky (1995) contends that the emphasis on independence and autonomy in rehabilitation is largely a reflection of the American ideal and dominates thinking to such an extent that its legitimacy is unquestioned. It has already been argued that independence and autonomy may not be appropriate for severely disabled or very frail individuals, and such considerations apply equally to differing ethnic and cultural groups. Greater attention to these areas is needed if equity and conceptual adequacy is to be achieved in rehabilitation.

McBride (1993) considers that chronic illness is a feminist issue, particularly as women live longer and are more likely to experience such conditions. Others also contend that gender, and particularly women's health, is a significant but neglected issue in rehabilitation and chronic illness (Howell, 1994; Masterson, 1994; Dangoor and Florian, 1994; Schaefer, 1995; Marris, 1996). Dangoor and Florian (1994) argue that women frequently suffer more disadvantage in areas such as resources, money and education and therefore have less at their disposal to deal with the demands of chronic illness. Others take a more existential stance, urging the creation of gender-sensitive theories (Howell, 1994) which recognise that women find it more difficult to validate the experience of chronic illness than do men, and may need additional help to rediscover their self-identity (Schaefer, 1995). For example Marris (1996) describes how women with chronic illness face an environment of oppression, and stresses the need to create a strong and positive disability culture. Women, she argues, face particular challenges when confronted with chronic illness as they tend to take their own health less seriously than the welfare of others. She highlights in particular the difficulties surrounding sexuality for disabled women, whose very identities tend to be associated more than do men's with this aspect of their lives. Gender issues are clearly relevant to rehabilitation but rarely figure as largely as they might in the wider literature and professional practice models. This appears to be an area requiring further research and theoretical development.

A different but no less important set of concerns surrounds the setting or location of rehabilitation. Emphasis within the rehabilitation literature is mainly placed on the early stages of the disablement process, with interventions primarily targeted on functional ability and the physical aspects of care. The onus is therefore on rehabilitation within hospital settings, yet the majority of care and rehabilitation occurs within the community, where the greatest deficits in service provision are apparent (Beardshaw, 1988; Baker et al, 1997). As Squires (1996) contends, rehabilitation takes place in a continuum of settings ranging from hospital through day hospital to out-patient departments and clinics, GPs' surgeries, the person's home and extending to residential and nursing home care. This diversity is not reflected in the literature. An extensive review by Lafferty (1996) suggests that the transfer of rehabilitation from hospital to the community is consistent with a number of policy objectives and assumed benefits including:

- the patient's natural desire to return home

- a reduction in the risks of hospitalisation

- better assessment of rehabilitation potential at home

- cost savings.

Despite such putative benefits, Lafferty argues that there is little quantifiable evidence of the superiority of rehabilitation in the patient's home and that scant attention has been given to the social, psychological and financial costs to patients and carers. Responding to Lafferty, Philp (1996) provides endorsement in principle for the move to community rehabilitation but cautions that this must not become community neglect. He advocates that the effectiveness of community alternatives should be established before the existing hospital infrastructure is dismantled.

Community rehabilitation is important for, as Mechanic (1995b) notes, there is a worldwide shift towards primary care, reinforced unequivocally in the UK in two recent White Papers (Secretary of State for Health, 1996b; 1996c). Indeed the White Paper on the Future of Primary Care (Secretary of State for Health, 1996b) reiterates many of the themes already covered in this review such as the creation of a seamless service, the need for better collaborative working and the forging of partnerships with patients and carers in order to enhance involvement and choice, especially in chronic disease.

Considerable remedial action is needed if such aims are to be realised and the fragmented and inconsistent service described by Beardshaw (1988) is to be improved. This will require a wider conceptualisation of rehabilitation which recognises its temporal nature and the fact that it spans not only disciplines and professions but also agencies, communities and ultimately society itself. For health professionals this means grappling with difficult issues about roles and responsibilities, and considering how services are organised and delivered (Barnes, 1993). As many problems faced by disabled people occur at times of transition across the 'seamless service', there is a need to design and test models for closer integration of primary and secondary care in chronic illness in order to enhance information exchange over and above that routinely occurring at discharge (Hickman et al, 1994). As so little attention has been paid to rehabilitation in community settings this represents one of a number of areas where the nursing role can be developed further.

NARROWING THE FOCUS: FROM MODELS TO MID-RANGE THEORIES AND CONCEPTS

5.1 Identifying recurring themes

Mirroring many of the arguments presented in this review, Price (1996) calls for *'recognition that the definitions of chronic illness, quality of life and comfort are legitimately the preserve of patients'*. Identifying common elements to aid assessment, he lists recurring themes in the literature on chronic illness: dealing with uncertainty; reconstructing self; managing regimes; managing relationships and a number of concepts related to the 'altered' body. Price advocates considering how these abstract ideas are interpreted by individual patients by using personal construct interviews. Although the concepts he cites are relevant they represent only a proportion of what might legitimately be described as 'recurring themes'. This chapter aims to identify a more comprehensive, although by no means exhaustive, selection of themes relevant rehabilitation in general and the nurse's role in particular. Many of these themes have their own extensive literature, so all that can be presented here is an overview, although selected concepts will be described in more detail to illustrate their potential application in a rehabilitation context. These have been purposively sampled to reflect orientations within the nursing literature.

5.2 Stress/coping and related concepts

One of the most widely applied theoretical perspectives can be broadly described as the stress-coping paradigm. A number of generalised models of the stress-coping relationship have been developed but the most adequate model is the transactional model of stress and coping which builds on the work of Lazarus and Folkman (Lazarus and Folkman, 1984; Folkman and Lazarus, 1985). Folkman and Lazarus (1985) define stress as *'a relationship between the person and the environment that is appraised by the person as relevant to his or her well-being and in which the person's resources are taxed or exceeded'*.

Within the transitional model it is not the objective components of events that determine their stressful nature but the manner in which they are perceived or interpreted by the individual. This is consistent with one of the dominant themes in the rehabilitation literature, the need to incorporate the subjective perceptions of disabled people. It is not surprising therefore that stress, coping and related concepts have been widely applied in the general literature on chronic illness, disability and rehabilitation, and more specifically in the nursing literature (Bailey and Clarke, 1989; Benner and Wruebel, 1989; Leidy et al, 1990). Speaking of chronic illness Lazarus (1992) suggests that stress and coping are now universally viewed as being microanalytic, contextual and process-orientated and argues that a primary focus for interventions is to help individuals adapt their coping responses to the stressors they face. After reviewing the literature over the last 25 years Lazarus (1993) argues that all coping strategies are *potentially* useful providing they are appropriate to the stressor itself. For example, if individuals can perceive events as a challenge rather than a threat, they experience less stress (Stoller and Pugliesi, 1989; Brown, 1993; Turnbull and Turnbull, 1993; Burr et al, 1994). Failing to acknowledge the importance of such individual interpretations is little short of *'professional self-deception'* (Lazarus, 1992).

Turnbull and Turnbull's (1993) definition of coping reflects the above orientation; these authors see the concept as referring to *'the things people do (acting and thinking) to increase a sense of wellbeing in their lives and to avoid being harmed by stressful events'*. Although numerous coping tactics can be employed, it is helpful to think of them as fitting into three categories:

- tactics aimed at the stressful event itself: problem-solving

- tactics aimed at the way an event is perceived: cognitive

- tactics aimed at reducing stress: relaxation.

As Pearlin and Scholler (1978) suggest, in this way coping behaviour may involve efforts to change or alleviate a difficult situation, alter or reduce a perceived threat, or manage the stress symptoms. Although the literature places great emphasis on problem-solving (Braithwaite, 1990; McKee et al, 1994; Ingebretsen and Solen, 1995) it is now more widely appreciated that individuals who employ a number of approaches and match their coping efforts to the stressor itself are likely to cope most effectively (Lazarus, 1993). It is of little use applying problem-solving efforts to a situation which cannot be changed, and while denial is often seen as a negative coping strategy a moderate degree may be helpful in chronic illness (Schussler, 1992). Similarly the ability to create *positive illusions* can be beneficial (Rolland, 1990; Guthrie and Harvey, 1994; Brown, 1993), indeed Brown (1993) considers a *high can-do* attitude essential to positive adaptation. Individuals with strong beliefs in themselves and optimistic attitudes appear to cope more effectively. This is consistent with the notion of *potency* which Ben-Sira (1989) sees as the ability either to deal with events or render them cognitively insignificant.

Similarly Brandstädter and colleagues (Brandstädter, 1995; Brandstädter and Greve, 1994; Brandstädter et al, 1993) argue that the balance between assimilative, accommodative and immunising strategies largely determines mental wellbeing in disability and illness. Individuals who continue to pursue unobtainable goals are more likely to suffer depression and related illnesses whereas those who can identify new but equally valued goals or see themselves as fortunate when compared to others are far less likely to have psychological problems. Related notions underpin the salutogenic model of health suggested by Antonovsky (1987) which has as one of its central constructs the idea of creating a sense of 'coherence'.

Although the above models are often presented as alternative conceptualisations, they reflect a general orientation permeating much of the literature on chronic illness and disability. This relates to the perceptual, interactional and dynamic nature of adjustment which relies upon subjective appraisal rather than objective reality. Such a model is not confined to the stress/coping literature: definitions of quality of life (Renwick and Brown, 1996) recognise the importance of a congruence between life conditions and hopes and expectations. McDaniel and Bach (1994) see quality of life as a key concept in rehabilitation nursing comprising four interrelated elements:

- the ability to set and achieve goals

- the ability to express feelings of contentment (or discontent)

- the ability to initiate and respond to change

- the ability to develop and maintain satisfying relationships.

Unfortunately, chronic illness and disability pose a number of threats to maintaining an acceptable quality of life; foremost among these are situations provoking uncertainty/unpredictability and powerlessness/helplessness.

Miller (1992a) suggests that a central focus for nursing in chronic illness is to maintain quality of life by sustaining and creating individuals' *power resources*, and develops a model arising from the views of patients and families. Powerlessness is defined as *the perception that one lacks the capacity or authority to act to affect an outcome* (Miller, 1992a) and Miller argues that chronic illnesses induce profound feelings of powerlessness as they affect multiple aspects of a patient's life and their demands are never completely eliminated. She believes a range of concepts such as control, helplessness and coping relate to powerlessness, while Stapleton (1992) asserts that a 'prototypical' nursing intervention plan comprises:

- modifying the environment

- helping the patient set realistic goals and expectations

- increasing patient knowledge

- increasing the sensitivity of health care providers and significant others

- encouraging verbalisation of feelings.

The same text discusses other potential nursing interventions including therapeutic use of the literature (Hobus, 1992), imagery (Stephens, 1992), facilitating behavioural change (Ryan, 1992), developing effective coping (Miller, 1992c), enhancing self-esteem (Miller, 1992d) and inspiring hope (Miller, 1992e). Miller (1992a) provides an overarching framework within which to consider a number of issues and presents powerlessness as a unique nursing diagnosis. However, she draws heavily on a wide range of theoretical orientations, particularly the coping literature and concepts such as locus of control.

5.2.1   Uncertainty

The importance of exerting an element of control is central to an understanding of a related area of the literature including concepts such as uncertainty and unpredictability. These figure prominently in both the general and nursing literature on rehabilitation (Felton et al, 1984; Robinson, 1988; Corbin and Strauss, 1988; Rolland, 1988; 1994; Mishel and Braden, 1988; Partridge and Johnston, 1989; Braden, 1990; Loveys, 1990; Cohen, 1993; Mishel, 1993; Schaefer, 1995; Marris, 1996).

Various 'types' of uncertainty have been postulated such as: *event, temporal, aetiologic, treatment, and prognostic* (Cohen, 1993) or *symptom, medication and diagnostic, and daily living* (Mishel, 1993) and it is widely acknowledged that reducing uncertainty is a key goal in rehabilitation (Mishel and Braden, 1988; Loveys, 1990; Braden, 1990; Cohen, 1993; Mishel, 1993) if individuals are to feel a sense of control and mastery (Felton et al, 1984; Partridge and Johnston, 1989; Dangoor and Florian, 1994).

Braden (1990) sees chronic illness as presenting a *'new learning condition'* and suggests there is a need to use a range of theories in order to help develop enabling skills. To achieve this Mishel (1993) contends that nurses must understand the tactics or *'illness schema'* developed by patients and families to deal with uncertainty. These appear to be conceptually similar to the notion of a *'trajectory projection'* suggested by Corbin and Strauss (1988). Interventions that assist patients in formulating an illness scheme include focusing on positive aspects of their situation and specifying and identifying controllable events (Mishel, 1993).

Cohen (1993) suggests that events around the time of diagnosis are particularly important as this is a time of *'rupture'* for patients but of *'closure'* for doctors. Nurses need to recognise patients' uncertainty and assist them to *'transform and reconstitute assumptive worlds'* (Cohen, 1993). The importance of diagnosis and the resulting range of practical and existential tasks have also been identified by others (Corbin and Strauss, 1988; 1991; 1992; Rolland, 1988; 1994) and there is potential for nurses to play a significant role in helping individuals understand and come to terms with their situation. Adequate information is essential if uncertainty is to be reduced (Strauss et al, 1984; Corbin and Strauss, 1988; 1991; Loveys, 1990) and, as will be highlighted in Section 6.2, many authors see patient education as one of the major nursing interventions in rehabilitative care.

5.3 Motivation

Other concepts consistent with an essentially psychological perspective on rehabilitation include motivation and encouragement. A number of authors suggest that motivation is the key to successful rehabilitation (Jackson, 1987; Kemp, 1988; 1993; Mosqueda, 1993; Guthrie and Harvey, 1994; Williams, 1994; Mulley, 1994; Mechanic, 1995b; Resnick, 1996). As with stress/coping, motivation has its own extensive literature and is variously interpreted and defined (Guthrie and Harvey, 1994). Seeking to impose some order on this disparate literature Guthrie and Harvey (1994) identify a number of theoretical orientations that have been applied:

- *goal setting models*: these include the patient and family in setting achievable goals. Ward and McIntosh's (1993) model epitomises this approach

- *self-sufficiency and control models*: these include concepts such as locus of control, learned helplessness

- *coping and appraisal models*: these are considered in some detail above

- *self-image models*: involve hope, optimism, the creation of possible futures (described below).

This consideration of motivation adopts an inclusive definition and subsumes a number of models already discussed. However, in identifying the core attributes which appear to transcend any particular theoretical orientation, Guthrie and Harvey (1994) suggest that the following are essential to maintain motivation:

- information, to reduce threat and restore control

- choice/goal setting (of optimistic rather than strictly realistic goals)

- attention to social and emotional needs, creating a new sense of self

- discouraging families from being over-protective

- creating a sense of hope and optimism

- providing a positive role model, for example a similarly disabled/ill person who has achieved success.

In contrast to Guthrie and Harvey's (1994) overview of motivation, Kemp (1988; 1993) develops a specific model. He argues that motivation is a frequently used but poorly defined concept, and to aid interpretation, presents a formula:

$$\text{Motivation} = \frac{\text{wants} \times \text{belief} \times \text{rewards}}{\text{risks/costs}}$$

Kemp (1993) believes that an assessment of wants and beliefs is important when *initiating* action, but that the balance between rewards and costs determines whether behavioural change is *maintained*. If someone wants something badly enough they will strive for it, but if the risks or costs outweigh the rewards, the behaviour will be discontinued. Kemp suggests that this balance is the key to successful rehabilitation, which reinforces the centrality of subjective perception and individual appraisal. Kemp (1993) argues that rehabilitation hinges on finding new goals or new ways of achieving old ones. However, as already highlighted the perceptions of patients and professionals are often at variance, and this applies equally to establishing motivational goals (Guthrie and Harvey, 1994).

Resnick (1996) in a qualitative study, identifies a number of patients that staff considered to lack motivation. However, when she interviewed these patients they perceived the failure to lie with staff who did not understand their needs. The patients felt that belief in themselves and in staff was an essential component of motivation and that this required staff to encourage them through kindness, humour and the identification of relevant goals – a relationship described as *'power with'*. Unfortunately patients often felt that staff dominated them and did not identify goals that patients valued or considered achievable, described as *'power over'* relationship. Authors such as Oliver (1993) argue that this is a manifestation of power differentials inherent in interactions between disabled people and professionals, an area which merits greater attention.

Adopting a broadly similar stance Beck (1994) talks of the need for *(en)couraging* as opposed to discouraging interventions in rehabilitation with the aim of rehabilitating the *will* in the face of medical passivity to chronic illness. This involves three levels:

- *I conceive*: creating the ability to see things as 'possible'

- *I can*: the creation of a sense of self-sufficiency

- *I will*: a commitment to action.

Again emphasis is placed on the 'I' component and as already noted the need to create a new sense of 'I' (self) is a prerequisite to successful adaptation (Beckmann and Ditlev, 1992). This orientation is reflected in the wider literature on rehabilitation and adaptation to chronic illness. Unfortunately interactions with health professions often do not acknowledge this (Charmaz, 1987) and Anderson (1991) suggests that nurses' interventions often heighten a devalued sense of self.

5.4 Psychosocial interventions

In addition to strategies designed to increase patients' motivation a range of other psychosocial interventions have been suggested, not all of which necessarily require the input of a psychologist or psychotherapist. These may include help with: grief and loss; disability counselling; breaking bad news; anxiety management; depression (Twinning, 1996) or: relaxation; focusing on pleasant events; cognitive restructuring; naming and responding to emotions; increasing knowledge of the disease process (Knight, 1996). With appropriate training nurses may have a role to play here (Sheppard, 1994a; 1994b; Hobus, 1992; Stephens, 1992). As well as psychological perspectives, Siegrist (1995) believes several mid-range sociological theories are useful to understanding a sense of self, and while space preludes a detailed consideration of these, a number of nursing related concepts and models are described briefly below.

A number of authors suggest that nurses are ideally placed to assist patients to reaffirm and re-establish their self-image and identity (Gullickson, 1993; Baker and Stern, 1993; Sheppard, 1994a; 1994b). This involves helping patients find meaning in their situation, identifying possibilities for control and promoting healing and personal growth that transcends the disease (Peace, 1996), which can be difficult, particularly in the early stages of illness/disability when patients may *'lose it'* if their suffering becomes unbearable (Dewar and Morse, 1995). Such individuals are often seen as difficult by nurses who fail to appreciate their emotional turmoil. A number of intrapersonal and interpersonal aspects of illness may become unbearable for patients and cause them to lose control, often resulting in verbal or physical aggression. Dewar and Morse (1995) argue that nurses should help patients to *'bear'* events and later to begin to manage them by, for example, learning to revalue personal qualities or develop new skills.

They advocate that caregivers (nurses) must appreciate events from the patient's perspective, and help to release tension or gain control by providing clear and understandable explanations and permitting choice. It is also suggested that 'losing it' occasionally can be therapeutic, allowing the expression of anger, hurt and pain, letting go of unrealistic hopes and creating new, more realistic goals. Such emotional expression and the modification of hope is crucial to successful rehabilitation, and should be an essential component of nurse education (Dewar and Morse, 1995).

'Losing it' (Dewar and Morse, 1995) gives explicit acknowledgement to the importance of affective responses to traumatic or chronic illness; two other such responses are chronic sorrow (Lindgren et al, 1992; Hainsworth et al, 1994) and guilt (Flannery, 1990). Chronic sorrow is not seen as pathological but rather as a normal response to chronic illness and disability which patients often need help to recognise and deal with (Lindgren et al, 1992; Hainsworth et al, 1994). Hainsworth et al argue that there are typically four patterns of response which are broadly consistent with the coping tactics described earlier (Section 5.2) and which provide a framework to assist nurses in helping patients recognise and deal with chronic sorrow:

- interpersonal, talking over worries and fears

- cognitive, reframing events and seeing them in a different light

- action, keeping active and busy

- emotional, giving vent to feelings.

Guilt is often a response to trauma and injury and is a pervasive emotion in family caregiving (Nolan et al, 1996). Flannery (1990) highlights the importance of nurses helping both patients and families acknowledge and address the guilt they may experience, and says that failure to deal with guilt can immobilise the whole family. She provides a model of how this may be achieved, using the acronym GUILT to identify the main stages:

Phase		Emotional response	
G	–	Grasping for reasons	*Hapless*
U	–	Unrealistic perceptions	*Helpless*
I	–	Immobilised by despair	*Hopeless*
L	–	Living reality	*Reframing*
T	–	Total resolution	(adapted from Flannery, 1990)

Flannery (1990) provides detailed guidelines to identify and respond to the above phases but at the heart of the model is the need to allow the expression of feeling, establish trust and begin to address the existence of guilt; state the reality of the situation so that reframing can begin; help patients and families predict the future and the likely consequences of the trauma/disease so that role changes can be identified; give specific direction to allow the exploration of options. Flannery's description of guilt typifies the value of mid-range theories that many argue represent the most useful form of knowledge for nursing (Nolan and Grant, 1994; Lenz et al, 1995; Levine, 1995).

Qualitative models of the illness experience developed from disabled people's accounts highlight the importance of existential and biographical components. This is reflected in the wider literature by concepts such as hope, hopelessness and spirituality. Barnard (1995) suggests that hope is an everyday concept in chronic illness but argues that it represents a *'boundary concept'* in the theoretical literature because it crosses a number of disciplines and paradigms and so does not belong to a well-defined intellectual tradition. However, hope is seen to epitomise the existential element of illness concerned with sustaining creativity in the face of adversity. Barnard (1995) believes that interventions should focus on *'remoralising'* individuals and that professionals must develop the *'empathetic witnessing'* skills needed to help disabled people make sense of and value their lives. Although Barnard (1995) is not writing from a nursing perspective the similarities between empathetic witnessing and concepts such as *'presencing'* (Benner, 1984) are clear. It is not surprising therefore that hope and hopelessness receive frequent mention in the nursing literature (Soeken and Carson, 1987; Miller, 1992b; Conwill, 1993; Farran et al, 1995; Morse and Doberneck, 1995). Miller (1992b) sees hope as a *'state of being'* comprising both generalised components (a perception that life is worth living) and particular elements directed towards specific goals. Morse and Doberneck (1995), however, argue that despite being frequently used, the concept remains poorly understood and is generally described in a way that is too abstract for practical application. They believe that hope is best conceived of as an active process sustained by setting realistic goals and expectations.

Other conceptualisations of hope take a more abstract perspective with it providing a link to the spiritual dimensions of illness and disability (Soeken and Carson, 1987; Hunt-Raleigh, 1992; Davies, 1994). Spirituality is not confined to religious faith but consists of those basic beliefs that positively affirm life (Soeken and Carson, 1987). A number of authors see spirituality as an essential component of nursing care in illness and disability but one that is inadequately addressed in training and practice (Soeken and Carson, 1987; Davies, 1994).

Sexuality is also an aspect of nursing care considered to be an important but neglected aspect of disability. It receives attention in areas such as spinal injury but is also considered to be of more general relevance (Rieve, 1989; Masterson, 1994; Marris, 1996). Rieve (1989), for example, advocates the Annon's (1976) model which uses the acronym PLISSIT to signify four levels or components of sexuality, each requiring increasingly specialised knowledge.

Permission   –   creating a climate which facilitates discussion of issues around sexuality

Limited **I**nformation – of a non-personal and generalised nature

Specific **S**uggestions   – relating to the sexual history of individual clients

Intensive **T**herapy   – requiring interventions from specialist counsellors

This, as will be discussed later (see Chapter 9), is a model that could be applied to other areas of nursing practice.

The foregoing all relate to the more diffuse, less tangible aspects of rehabilitation and the desirability of viewing chronic illness and disability from a health and wellness perspective has already been highlighted (Milz, 1992; RCN, 1994). In operationalising this approach Lindsey (1996) outlines a model of *'health within illness'* which comprises six themes which unite many of the concepts discussed in this section. These themes highlight the importance of:

- honouring self and respecting who you are

- maintaining relationships and reciprocity

- seeing illness as presenting a challenge and opportunity

- transcending the illness

- celebrating a life with illness, a process which reinforces the value of being alive

- recognising the spiritual aspects of illness.

Lindsey (1996) believes that nurses have a key role in facilitating achievement of the above aims but argues that there is a need for a *'fundamental transformation in their philosophical perspective'* which moves nursing care beyond a simple problem-solving framework. This reinforces the importance of the interpersonal dynamic in rehabilitation nursing, in particular the need for nurses to appreciate and value patients' subjective experiences. Lamb and Stempel (1994) see the formation of a long-term relationship as essential and contend that a significant nursing task is to assist patients to become *'insider experts'*, capable of being their own care managers.

Lamb and Stempel describe three interrelated and hierarchical elements which are central to positive adaptation: *affective; cognitive and behavioural components*. The affective element is a prerequisite to subsequent stages and involves establishing trust between nurse and patient, and cannot be achieved until the patient is satisfied that the nurse knows and understands him or her as an individual. The second element is termed *'working'* and concerns a cognitive shift in perception towards redefinition of self as complete and valuable. Only then can the behavioural element *'changing'* be considered, when the patient is both able to help him- or her-self and accept help from others. In addition to their technical expertise, Lamb and Stempel (1994) describe a number of other nursing roles including: monitoring; co-ordinating; teaching and enabling. These and other potential roles will be considered in greater detail in Section 6.2.

5.4.1   The family

As noted earlier, families are also central to rehabilitation and family nursing has emerged as a significant orientation within nursing generally and rehabilitation in particular. Robinson (1995) argues for the need to identify a common nursing language with respect to families and to specify in greater detail what nurses *do* to orient them. While this might be some way off, the discourse of family nursing has permeated rehabilitation literature (Gillies, 1988; Knafl and Deatrick, 1990; Shaw and Halliday, 1992; Woods et al, 1993; Stetz et al, 1994; Weeks and O'Connor, 1994; Donnelly, 1995).

Gillies (1988) applies the concept of *'role insufficiency'* to families and argues that when family members take on new caregiving roles, the expectations of such roles must be clarified and the tasks or components delineated; this requires appropriate information, training and advice. Yet this rarely occurs, as was amply demonstrated in the literature previously reviewed (Section 4.3), and remains a considerable deficit within nursing practice. Knafl and Deatrick (1990) identify the importance of understanding families' *'management style'*, while Shaw and Halliday (1992) suggest that families require help if they are to evolve and meet the demands they face. Others believe that families need to have hope in the future and to see their situation as manageable (Weeks and O'Connor, 1994; Stetz et al, 1994). This orientation towards the family is also apparent in a number of related disciplines including medicine.

> *'The family perspective in health care is part of an intellectual and technological movement towards holistic and ecosystemic approaches to medicine that conceptually unite mind and body and consider people within their particular social contexts.'* (Bloch, 1993 pvii)

Bloch (1993) considers a family perspective to be part of a reorientation of medicine in chronic illness and disability which recognises the value of multiple inputs including those of general and specialist nurses. As previously suggested, Rolland's (1988; 1994) family systems illness model provides the sort of comprehensive framework from which nursing would benefit. However, irrespective of the family model applied, Rolland argues that the concepts of transaction and interaction underpin all systems approaches. This once again reinforces the dynamic and changing nature of rehabilitative care and this fluidity has considerable implications for developing the nurse's role.

REHABILITATION: IDENTIFYING THE DIMENSIONS OF THE NURSE'S CONTRIBUTION

6.1   Rethinking rehabilitation

Consensus as to a definition of rehabilitation has proved elusive (RCP, 1986; Tallis, 1992) and searching for one may be something of a chimera, as the concept is still evolving (Renwick and Friefield, 1996). It has been described as both a process and an achievement (Vreede, 1988) or alternatively as an attitude rather than a process (Mosqueda, 1993). Despite such differences in emphasis, however, there is widespread agreement that rehabilitation is a multifaceted and multidimensional activity incorporating a range of perspectives (disabled person, family carer, professional) across a number of phases (for example, crisis, chronic and terminal) addressing consequences at differing levels (impairment, disability, handicap) with interventions ranging from the individual through the family to community, society and the environment.

This more holistic orientation is reflected in some recent definitions such as that suggested by Pawlson (1994) who sees the aim of rehabilitation as being:

'... to secure for patients the best alternative future as defined by the patient, given their current status; the possible alternative interventions and the possibility of the interventions success in achieving the optimal state.' (p58)

Although broader than traditional medical definitions this involves a number of contingencies, so while the *'alternative future'* may be defined by the patient the range of *'possible alternative interventions'* is likely to remain the professional preserve, as is a consideration of their success. Here authors such as Oliver (1993) would argue that professionals exercise their unequal power. It seems reasonable to conclude that this broader vision of rehabilitation will not be realised until the range of possible interventions and consequent definitions of success are extended. Yet in the present period of financial retrenchment economic concerns are likely to exert an ever greater influence, as illustrated by Symington's (1994) perception of the aim of rehabilitation:

'... to reduce the burden of disability and handicap in society and to do so in ways that not only improve the quality of life of the disabled and handicapped person but also reduce the costs to society.' (p13)

If this is considered as a pattern of discourse it is interesting to note that quality of life is neatly sandwiched between the *burden* of disability and handicap and the need to reduce its *costs*. This general orientation to rehabilitation is manifest in approaches such as that advocated by Ward and McIntosh (1993) which, although putatively concerned with the subjective impact of disease and disadvantage, casts rehabilitation primarily within a *'functionally orientated framework'* based on establishing goals which are capable of objective, preferably quantifiable, verification. Although in a world of finite resources difficult decisions have to be made, the much-vaunted subjective perceptions of patients are unlikely to receive the priority they merit unless this emphasis is countered. Furthermore calls to extend the range of appropriate outcomes to areas such as reassurance, empathy and the reduction of uncertainty (Fitzpatrick, 1996) will struggle to gain other than tacit recognition when faced with arguments about the need to specify the relationship between the *'dose'* of rehabilitation and the *'response'* of the patient (Grainger et al, 1996). Therefore as Renwick and Friefield (1996) assert *'despite the higher order goal of enhancing quality of life, most interventions are focused on increasing function'.*

Dutton (1995), writing from a therapy perspective, believes that a consequence of the physical orientation towards rehabilitation is that psychological aspects are seldom explicitly acknowledged and become *'underground work'*. Here lies one of the greatest challenges for the nursing role in rehabilitation for, as Sheppard (1994a; 1994b) suggests, many nursing interventions are subtle and invisible and until they achieve a higher profile, greater recognition (from within and outside the profession) and explicit attention in the educational preparation of nurses progress cannot be made. This means considering whether there is potential for a more extensive nursing role in rehabilitation and what form such a role could take: generic, specialist or both; what range of skills and knowledge are required; and what barriers must be addressed.

Within a UK context commentators such as Sheppard (1994a; 1994b) and Waters (1996) believe that nurses should play a significant role in rehabilitation and the publication of standards of practice by the Royal College of Nursing (1994) reaffirms this. However, as described earlier (see Section 2.2), the current nursing role is very much secondary, largely being confined, as Waters (1996) notes, to *'general maintenance and carry-on'* functions with a specialist role accorded in such areas as promotion of continence and maintenance of skin integrity. Even adopting this restricted definition nurses often lack the necessary skills and knowledge to fulfil their responsibilities within a general rehabilitative context, and this is compounded by the fact that most nurses either cannot articulate their role clearly or do not see themselves as having a role, perceiving rehabilitation as the responsibility of the therapy disciplines (Walker, 1995; Johnson, 1995; Waters, 1996; Waters and Luker, 1996). This raises the fundamental question of whether there is (or could be) a generalised nursing role in rehabilitation or if this sphere should be confined to specialist areas such as cardiac rehabilitation or spinal injury.

Sheppard (1994a; 1994b) believes that rehabilitation of older and/or chronically ill people represents the nursing challenge of the 1990s, but if this is to be realised current practice in both hospital and community settings must improve. As numerous authors have attested, one of the distinguishing characteristics of chronic illnesses is their temporal nature and the likelihood that chronically ill and disabled people will have frequent contact with the health services, including periods of hospitalisation. Beardshaw (1988) argues that disabled people are poorly catered for, particularly in hospital, and that such difficulties are primarily attributable to their interactions with nurses. Similarly, in a community setting, recent studies highlight that although disabled people would value an ongoing relationship with nurses this is rarely achieved (NOP, 1996; Baker et al, 1997). The increasing numbers of frail older people and the shift in emphasis towards primary care provide a good case that there *must* be an increasing role for nurses in rehabilitation in both general and specialised settings.

The American literature is unequivocal on this point and considers that few areas of practice have so bright a future as rehabilitation (Preston, 1994) whether in generic or specialist practice (Stryker, 1996; Hoeman, 1996). This is seen to include acute care and chronic illness, with the latter being described as the *'task of the future'* (Funk et al, 1993), representing a domain in the ascendancy lying at the heart of nursing (McBride, 1993). However, even in the US, where rehabilitation has been a recognised area of nursing practice for longer, there is still seen to be a need to achieve greater prominence (Purk, 1993), better role clarity (Gibbons et al, 1995) and improved educational preparation (Hermann and Bays, 1994; Gonthier and Habel, 1994). Before rehabilitation nursing in the UK can flourish, therefore, there is a need for a clearly articulated vision. Although it may not currently be possible precisely to articulate such a vision, as a result of the initial review some clearer signposts can be suggested.

6.2   Beyond physical care

Nursing should recognise a role in rehabilitation which extends beyond physical care. However, recent debates still seem dominated by such an orientation. Gale and Gaylard (1996) recognise the fundamental role of nursing in restoring health, but proceed to describe rehabilitation in the following way:

> *'Assisting patients to overcome their handicaps, by helping them to return function to a part of the body or by optimising the use of remaining abilities, is the essence of rehabilitation ... the underlying philosophy of contemporary nursing is that care is based on planning and using skills that prevent deterioration or restore physical function immediately the patient is admitted to the ward or referred to the community team. Some have termed this rehabilitative nursing care.'* (p144)

Although the prevention of deterioration and the restoration of physical functioning are key components of rehabilitative nursing they cannot provide a complete definition. A logical extension of the above definition is a return to the nursing role in rehabilitation as described by Andrews (1987):

> *'Others have suggested that nurses could take on the basic rehabilitation work, thereby leaving the trained therapists free to carry out highly specialised rehabilitation techniques. Nurses are in a particularly suitable position to take on the general rehabilitation training of patients since they are responsible for the management of patients throughout the 24-hour period and spend more time with patients than any other professional group.'* (p15)

It is hard to argue with the above sentiments as nurses *do* spend more time with patients than any other group. However, this not only affords the opportunity to conduct 'basic rehabilitation work' but also to address the affective, cognitive, biographical and existential aspects of care consistently identified as essential components of rehabilitation.

Waters' (1996) conceptualisation of the nursing role in the form of a matrix with general maintenance, specialist and carry-on roles along one axis and patient education, health promotion, tissue viability, continence, dressing, mobility and personal hygiene along the other better reflects a more holistic approach but perhaps fails to capture the more subtle dimensions of the multidimensional role she advocates.

The RCN (1994) places an onus on health and wellbeing in rehabilitation, rather than illness and disability and although a definition of rehabilitation is not provided, it is recognised as *'a complex process involving a variety of people in helping the client and his family to make tremendous adjustments'*. In making such adjustments it is advocated that clients be co-manager, taking control of their own health. It is argued that this will mean nurses focusing on health promotion, utilising a suitable model and possessing knowledge and skills in a number of areas of assessment including: tissue viability, neurological observations, continence, functional ability, behavioural, psychological and emotional factors and health or related previous experiences. Complementing these aspects of care are skills in counselling and communication which include acknowledging and recognising when *'clients, carers, herself (the nurse) and colleagues'* may need specialist help. This approach is consistent with the graded hierarchy of interventions suggested by Rieve (1989) as applying to sexuality (see PLISSIT, Section 5.4) and Twinning (1996) about psychological interventions generally. The concept of basic skills being available to all nurses with specialist skills being developed by some is consistent with the present emphasis on specialist and advanced practice.

As might be anticipated, broader conceptualisations of the nurse's role are apparent in the American literature; Rieve's (1989) definition is a typical example:

'Rehabilitation nurses are concerned with persons with disabilities and provide comfort and therapy, promote health-conducive adjustment, support the individual's adaptive capabilities and promote achievable independence.' (p265)

The above definition recognises that nurses provide a multifaceted contribution to the rehabilitation process. Of all the nursing roles, an educative input is one of the most frequently cited, even by non-nurses (Strauss et al, 1984; Strauss and Corbin, 1988; Brillhart and Stewart, 1989; Thurgood, 1990; Lamb and Stempel, 1994; Preston, 1994; Sheppard, 1994a; 1994b; Hoeman, 1996; Waters, 1996). Indeed many see this role as the most important nursing contribution to rehabilitation. Education is seen to extend beyond simply giving information, to include helping patients reintegrate their lives (Coates and Boore, 1995). The importance of this was stressed some years ago by Strauss et al (1984) who, in a wide-ranging analysis of the care of chronically ill and disabled people in the US, identified a shift away from a medically dominated approach towards one in which nurses played a major teaching role. This role, according to the authors, should not be restricted to formal teaching but should involve a reciprocal relationship in which nurses learn from patients by giving explicit recognition and reinforcement to the 'work' that patients and families engage in. With such emphasis on an educative role, it is not surprising that considerable store is given to the acquisition of appropriate learning theory (Jackson, 1987; Brillhart and Stewart, 1989; Keith and Lipsey, 1993; Preston, 1994; Hoeman, 1996); Brillhart and Stewart (1989) suggest that rehabilitation nurses must be capable of delivering appropriate education starting at admission and involving all members of the rehabilitation team, particularly family carers, in both one to one and group contexts. An educative role certainly seems to be one of the perceived core competencies of rehabilitation nurses.

In addition to the physical components of care and the above instructional and educative elements, numerous other roles have been described and a composite of these is presented in Table 6.1. These suggestions are certainly expansive but the inherent risk of such inclusive frameworks is that they require such varied knowledge and skills that they are beyond the ability of any one individual. Many of the roles are also at such a level of generality that they are open to numerous and varied interpretations. One aspect that this review has brought into sharp relief is that although the application of multiple concepts to rehabilitation practice is advocated, most of these concepts are poorly defined. As noted earlier there is *always* tension between the very specific definitions needed for measurement purposes and the sort of vague exhortations that perpetuate 'reborn certainties'. There is a need to acknowledge such tensions and to begin to address them.

The notion of tightly specified operational definitions almost seems anathema to the individualised, contextual and dynamic aspects of rehabilitation highlighted throughout this review, yet they may be preferable to the rather trite and vague sentiments that nurses frequently call upon when defining their role. If nursing seriously intends to claim a unique role within rehabilitation that transcends general maintenance, a few specialist functions (continence, skin integrity) and a carry-on role, the profession must begin to articulate what this is. With respect to Table 6.1, this means bringing greater precision to bear. If the nurse is an enabler, *what* is being enabled? If the nurse is a co-ordinator or organiser, *who* or *what* is being co-ordinated and organised and are they aware of it? Underpinning many of the difficulties inherent in a teamwork philosophy is a failure to understand the role of other team members, compounded by communication problems occasioned in large measure by the use of implicit professional

Waters 1987	Corbin and Strauss 1991	Hymovich and Hagopian 1992	Brillhart and Sills 1994	Lamb and Stempel 1994	Hoeman 1996
Risk taker	Direct care	Establish/maintain trust	Caregiver	Technical expert	Educator
Enabler	Teach	Provide support/guidance	Counsellor	Monitoring	Counsellor
Healer	Counsel	Provide information	Collaborator	Coordinating	Care manager
Achiever	Make referrals	Provide anticipatory guidance	Educator	Teaching	Researcher
Befriender	Make arrangements	Facilitate stress reduction	Communicator	Enabling	Advocate
Imagination (use of)	Monitor	Facilitate self-care	Manager		Enabler and facilitator
Love (giver of moderated)		Facilitate access to resources	Staff developer		Teacher
Independence (facilitator of)		Modify attitudes			Expert practitioner
Treatment (giver of)		Assess all family members			Team member
Adviser		Provide direct care			
Teacher		Collaborate with others			
Intimate care (giver of)					
Organiser					
Nurturer					

Table 6.1: Some suggested components of the nursing role in rehabilitation and chronic illness

theories and values. Overcoming these tensions requires as a minimum greater specification of roles so that these can be shared, debated or at least acknowledged, even if a consensus proves elusive. Furthermore, it is not possible to provide an appropriate educational preparation based on the level of generality apparent in much of the debate about the nurse's role in rehabilitation. Achieving greater specificity along a number of dimensions is a key task in elucidating more clearly the nursing contribution to rehabilitation within the multidisciplinary team.

6.3   Towards a more extensive nursing contribution

One of the main challenges in completing this review has been the breadth and diversity of the literature and the necessity to differentiate the rhetoric of rehabilitation from the reality as described by disabled and chronically ill people and their carers. There now seems widespread agreement that rehabilitation is multifaceted and relevant across a number of contexts and situations. It can no longer be seen to be confined to the acute and sub-acute stages of illness, but must include preventive measures aimed at reducing the incidence of disability and trauma and extend beyond impairment to address disability and handicap. The legitimate sphere of intervention therefore ranges from the molecular through to the societal, and includes the organ or system, individual, family and community. Furthermore, whether for altruistic or ideological reasons, the language of partnership and empowerment is pervasive. It is therefore not surprising that the concept of rehabilitation defies easy definition.

In marked contrast to the above stand the accounts of disabled people and their carers, from which emerges the picture of a health care system that, by and large, is still dominated by the *'acute simple disease model'* (Pawlson, 1994), with a rehabilitative ethos which reflects the short-term rather than the long-term model (Robinson, 1988). The discourse of rehabilitation is frankly contradictory in espousing the value of patient involvement and the importance of subjective perceptions while simultaneously refining quantifiable outcome measures and critical pathways.

It is argued here that nurses, rather than as Robinson (1988) suggests therapists, are in the ideal position to build a bridge between short-term and long-term rehabilitation and to marry the objective with the subjective. Certainly there is an hiatus here and the present flux in the health services provides the ideal opportunity to fill it. Nursing therefore may wish to be proactive and seize this opportunity, not simply because it is expedient and opportune, but rather because the nursing profession is best placed to do so. As Beardshaw (1988) notes a coherent and organised framework to address the needs of chronically ill and disabled people is lacking, a contention which has been recently reinforced (NOP, 1996; Baker et al, 1997). One of the reasons that nursing lays claim to a major role in rehabilitation in a hospital context is that they are the only group providing 24-hour care. It could also be argued that of all professional groups, nursing is the only one with potential input at all stages or phases of illness. As noted above, however, if this potential is to be realised greater specificity as to the interventions nurses might provide and how they may best be prepared educationally to deliver them is needed. The following section utilises the ICIDH framework to suggest how the nurse's role in rehabilitation might be expanded.

6.4   Expanding the nursing role

Hoeman (1996) contends that rehabilitation nursing is concerned with lifelong care transitions and incorporates primary prevention, acute, sub-acute and tertiary interventions. It involves both generic and specialist components (Stryker, 1996) and is delivered in all contexts and settings (Preston, 1994). This reinforces the assertion that nurses can lay the best claim to provide both 24-hour coverage and a relevant input in all phases of rehabilitation. The purpose here is to suggest what the nursing role might be when viewed through differing sets of theoretical lenses.

As noted earlier, the ICIDH stimulated considerable debate about the purpose of rehabilitation and helped to reinforce the limitations of the medical model. Its most significant contribution has been to focus attention on the consequences of disease so that the social impact of disability is a legitimate area of professional concern. It therefore seems appropriate to begin a discussion of the nurse's role in rehabilitation using the ICIDH as a basis for analysis. To recapitulate, the ICIDH consists of four elements representing a temporal but not necessarily a causal ordering:

Disease/Disorder → Impairment → Disability → Handicap

or Trauma (from Badley, 1995 p55).

As other authors have suggested, rehabilitation, although traditionally associated with the disability component of this model, can legitimately be seen to begin at the level of primary prevention to reduce or prevent disease or trauma (Hershenson, 1990; Livneh, 1995). In this context, interventions are largely in the domain of public health and interestingly both Livneh and Hershenson see no role for nurses at this level. However, within the UK, public health has been the subject of considerable recent attention, highlighting in particular the role of the health visitor (Cowley, 1995; SNMAC, 1995). The influential SNMAC (1995) report stresses the importance of all nurses, midwives and health visitors contributing both to individual health and to that of communities, via community development and alliances which facilitate people taking greater control of their own health. Such a role is consistent with major government policy statements over recent years, and the SNMAC (1995) report recommends that the National Boards *give special attention to public health content and intended learning outcomes when approving education programmes*. If the broad definition of rehabilitation suggested by authors such as Henshenson (1990) is accepted, there is clearly a major role for nurses and health visitors. Even if this preventive role is seen to be outwith the domain of rehabilitation, the health needs of chronically ill and disabled people are not, and, as will be discussed later in this section, health visitors may have a major role to play here.

Although much of the emphasis within this review has been on disability and handicap, Tallis (1992) argues that the future of rehabilitation lies in efforts to cure or reverse impairment. He warns against what he terms *'misplaced holism'* believing that technological and other advances will open up new possibilities to address impairment. There is both logic and merit in his argument – most people, given an option, would choose to be cured. However, this remains a goal to aspire to rather than current reality, so a wider conceptualisation of rehabilitation is still needed.

The acute phase of illness or trauma (impairment) presents many opportunities for a nursing role. Cope and Sundance's (1995) framework permits a detailed consideration of what the nurse's contribution might be. These authors outline a six-stage model, each with their associated outcomes:

0   physiologic instability

I   physiologic stability

II   physiologic maintenance

III residential integration

IV   community reintegration

V   productive activity.

The above authors argue that the most important goal of rehabilitation is to achieve physiologic stability. This has been achieved when *'all major medical issues have been resolved to the extent that discharge from an acute hospital is clinically appropriate'*. As this model was developed in a US context this criterion may not be entirely applicable in the UK, but the level of physiologic stability is nevertheless concerned with acute management of trauma and stress. Building on this framework Sundance and Cope (1995) see the nursing role at level I as comprising primarily efforts to prevent secondary complications across a range of fronts including: wound care; bowel and bladder management; joint protection; skin management; airway management; feeding and nutritional programme and pulmonary toilet. Such management would probably be undertaken in an intensive therapy unit (ITU) in the UK and clearly requires a range of knowledge and skills, some of which may be relevant to generic practice but most of which are associated with more intensively orientated areas of care.

The shift in emphasis from impairment to disability may, for example, be signalled by transferring the patient from ITU to a general ward. It is during this transitionary period and subsequently up until the point of discharge from hospital that the nurse's role in rehabilitation is traditionally described, and the general maintenance and carry-on functions emerge. In suggesting a more specific nursing role, it is important not to lose sight of the need to maintain physical integrity and to reinforce progress in the functional domain of rehabilitation, in addition to providing expert care in areas such as continence and the maintenance of skin integrity.

Kelly-Hayes (1996) argues that if nurses are to make an optimal contribution to rehabilitation, they must be able to base their assessments and evaluations on something other than their own perceptions. She believes that functional assessment is integral to rehabilitative care and contends that nurses should be able to discuss knowledgeably the relative merits of differing assessment tools. This would not only help to articulate the nursing role but, as such indices are frequently used by other disciplines, would provide a basis for better multidisciplinary dialogue and communication. It is therefore important that nurses understand the principles underpinning scale construction and know the commonly used indices. A basic appreciation might be gained at qualification with more detailed knowledge being developed later.

However, while there is obviously a role for nurses in the physical care of patients during the transition from impairment to disability, other areas are also important. In outlining a prototypical *'critical pathway'* for the early stages of rehabilitation Bryant (1995) suggests that nursing roles should include, in addition to physical care, the maintenance of a safe environment, an assessment of the patient's affect and the initiation of patient and family teaching, including a consideration of coping and adjustment strategies. A more proactive nursing role in patient and carer education and assessment is required in the UK, both in a rehabilitative context and more generally relating to the care of disabled and chronically ill people in hospital. As already highlighted a number of models and mid-range theories are available, and these should be reflected in basic educational programmes.

In terms of the ICIDH the issue of handicap has posed the greatest challenge, not only in achieving an agreed definition but also in terms of service developments (Badley, 1995). This is a reflection of the distance, in conceptual terms, between handicap and the traditional medical approach to health care. For disabled people however, handicap, representing the social consequences of disease or trauma, is of great significance. Here the biographical and existential components figure prominently and current deficits in health care are brought into most sharp relief.

Working with disabled people and their carers to address handicap is complex, subtle and involves establishing a relationship of trust (Thorne, 1993; Lamb and Stempel, 1994;

Hoeman, 1996). The ICIDH presents a rather neat and over-orderly impression of impairment → disability → handicap, but this does not mean that interventions cannot be provided concurrently. As soon as impairment occurs, consideration of all aspects of rehabilitation should begin. For example, following traumatic injury, mid-range theories might be used to consider the transition from victim to patient to disabled person (Morse and O'Brien, 1995) and to identify those *'unbearable'* incidents in which individuals may *'lose it'* (Dewar and Morse, 1995). However, as Lamb and Stempel (1994) suggest, before patients can begin to redefine self and *'change'* in terms of learning to help themselves and accept help from others they must *'bond'* with their professional care providers and see them as *'insider experts'*.

This is when efforts to create a sense of *'health within illness'* (Lindsey, 1996) should begin. However, to be successful nurses need to transform their philosophical perspective away from simple problem-solving models (Lindsey, 1996). This does not mean that problem-solving is always inappropriate, but that it is only one of a range of possible interventions. If nurses are to expand their role in rehabilitation they must be able to specify what interventions they promote and why. Fortunately a range of options is present in the literature, any of which would probably lead to an improvement in current practice. Central to all such approaches is the creation of a strong and positive relationship between disabled people, their families and health care professionals. Fundamentally there is a need to acknowledge and validate the subjective reality of disabled people and work with them to envisage possible futures. Attention to the biographical and existential consequences of disease or trauma are therefore vital.

Although this involves a subtle period of relationship-building, a number of more concrete interventions can also be offered, such as dealing with guilt (Flannery, 1990) or sexuality (Rieve, 1989); helping to reduce uncertainty by building positive coping strategies (Mishel, 1993); enhancing decision-making skills (Loveys, 1990); and seeing chronic illness and disability as a new learning condition (Braden, 1990). Complementing the existential components there is a major role in teaching and learning, providing information, working to understand and help *'shape'* the illness trajectory (Corbin and Strauss, 1991; 1992). The area of handicap provides the opportunity to shift the focus from illness and disability to health and wellness (RCN, 1994) which will mean overcoming the present preoccupation with physical care, important as this aspect may be.

Although there is greater recognition of the importance of handicap as a major focus of intervention in rehabilitation this is only beginning to permeate practice. Davies (1995) found that nurses still focus on the physical aspects of care, equating physical independence with wellness, and presents a health promotion model for use in rehabilitation which might help improve current practice. Major and significant roles with family carers are also relevant at this time, and this is an area of practice in which there is considerable potential for nurses to take a lead role (Nolan et al, 1996).

A number of authors argue that the situation of disabled people will not improve until professional training is reorientated (Beardshaw, 1988; Morse and Johnson, 1991; Barnitt and Pomeroy, 1995; Peters, 1995). Fulford (1996) feels that a balanced curriculum should include not only the traditional focus on facts and disease but also perspectives on values and experience. On the basis of the initial review it became apparent that there is also a need for considerable emphasis not only on areas such as health promotion and teaching skills, but also *how* these relate to chronically ill and disabled people. Such a reorientation of the professional psyche needs to permeate all health disciplines, particularly medicine, and considerable work remains to be done in this area (Ricke, 1992; Lafaille, 1992). Simply rebalancing the nursing curriculum is likely to be insufficient; for real change to occur nurses need a greater appreciation of the needs of chronically ill and disabled people and the skills to deliver differing interventions.

The literature suggests that even in the physical components of care, where nurses are accorded 'expert' status by others, practitioners often lack the necessary knowledge to fulfil such a role adequately. A rebalancing of the curriculum should not therefore be at the expense of such components but needs to include at least a basic understanding of counselling and other skills.

The literature indicates that the nurse's current role in rehabilitation in the UK, limited as it is, is confined mainly to hospital settings. Addressing the issue of handicap necessarily extends this considerably, particularly if it is accepted that rehabilitation is not a finite but an on-going process. If chronically ill and disabled people are to be treated as 'well', then attention to their needs in the community is a prerequisite, and the influence of external factors is particularly relevant.

Attention to external factors which act as barriers to rehabilitation (Mechanic, 1995a) means addressing societal attitudes to disabled people and attending to physical limitations imposed by the built environment. Given the renewed policy thrust towards public health there is a potentially significant role for community health care nurses in this area, including district nurses and practice nurses, but particularly health visitors. There is scope for the introduction of specific training or counselling with disabled people and their carers as suggested by Braden (1993) who adapted a mid-range theory of self-help and devised a training programme for nurses working in the community.

A major conclusion of Beardshaw's (1988) extensive review of services for disabled people is the lack of a coherent system, confirmed by recent studies (Robinson and Batstone, 1996; Baker et al, 1997). Beardshaw (1988) identifies the need for far greater co-ordination, a role she considered the health visitor might fulfil. Interestingly Thorne (1993) in a US study, reaches almost identical conclusions, suggesting that if the health care needs of chronically ill and disabled people are to be addressed adequately, two significant barriers must be ameliorated: the dominant biomedical ideology; and the *complex, inefficient and frustrating* organisation of services, which fail to reflect the needs of chronically ill people. Thorne (1993) concludes that *'an important element missing from health care for chronic illness is, therefore, the co-ordinating function'*. She argues that patients and families find nurses' input particularly useful here and suggests, as does Beardshaw (1988), that nurses could fulfil this important but neglected co-ordination function. This is consistent with the role suggested by Corbin and Strauss (1991; 1992) as an arranger and referrer. This is not simply an administrative task but requires detailed knowledge of both the health and social care system and the needs of individual patients.

On the basis of the above it is contended that community health care nurses in general, but health visitors in particular, could play a considerably expanded role in community rehabilitation, especially in terms of public health. Others, such as district nurses, also have an important role in working with disabled people and their carers on a range of fronts including enhancement of coping and adjustment to illness or disability.

At a more generalised level nurses need to influence the politics of disability and chronic illness. Authors such as Oliver (1993), Thorne (1993) and Marris (1996) highlight the power differentials inherent in interactions between disabled people and both health care providers and society. The nursing literature is replete with notions of advocacy, empowerment and partnership, as are recent policy documents on the future of health care (Secretary of State for Health, 1996a; 1996b; 1996c). Making a reality of these ideals requires concerted action to raise the profile of chronically ill and disabled people at all levels of the health care system. Nursing can play a significant role in this respect but to do so adequately, nurses need greater awareness of how the needs of disabled people are perceived by the individuals concerned. They also need to play a more politically active role. Preparation for practice at all levels should reflect this.

In this section we have used the ICIDH as an analytic device to highlight a number of areas in which the current nursing role in rehabilitation might be expanded. Other frameworks could legitimately have been employed for the same purpose, for example, the concept of 'work' advocated by many authors would have been useful (Corbin and Strauss, 1991; 1992; Thorne, 1993). Similarly Mumma and Nelson (1996) describe a number of models for theory-based rehabilitation nursing including: client-centred models (focusing on disability/culture/family); setting-centred models (acute care/long-term care/community/home care); provider-centred models (primary care/care management/nurse managed care/independent practice); and collaborative practice models (multidisciplinary teams/interdisciplinary teams/transdisciplinary teams) which, although developed in the US, provide a most useful heuristic framework. Social models of disability are also relevant (Oliver, 1993; Finkelstein and Stuart, 1996).

It could be argued that one of these other frameworks *should* have been used, as they might better represent the orientations of disabled people by presenting viable alternatives to the existing medical dominance. However, while there is a need for substantial changes to rehabilitation practice, success is likely to require a delicate balance between evolution and revolution. The use of the ICIDH is therefore felt to be appropriate for two reasons. First, rehabilitation cannot be considered in isolation from acute, curative models, as the acute simple disease model and the chronic complex illness model (Pawlson, 1994) need to co-exist, each being legitimate in the appropriate context; the ICIDH allows a consideration of this relationship. Second, if rehabilitation practice is to improve, nurses may need to *'lead the charge'* but cannot achieve success alone. The essence of rehabilitation is teamwork, and other team members must be party to any significant reorientation of current roles. Frameworks from the sociological or nursing literature, while potentially useful, are not part of mainstream medical discourse. Although the ICIDH has yet to penetrate the further reaches of medicine it is a more integral part of professional vocabulary, and therefore provides the most appropriate vehicle with which to engage in meaningful multidisciplinary dialogue.

6.5 Constructing a framework

In respect of nursing there is a need to construct a framework to help elucidate both rehabilitation and the potential nursing contribution. We attempt this here. On the basis of the initial review of the literature on the models, theories and concepts of rehabilitation and the current nursing role in rehabilitation a number of dimensions were identified. These are summarised in Figure 6.1, and described in more detail below.

Henderson (1980) saw the *'unique'* contribution of nurses to rehabilitation as relating primarily to their 24-hour, seven-day input. We consider, however, that this is a rather limited basis upon which to lay claim to a unique role. While nurses do provide a 24-hour, seven-day service (although this is debatable in some environments) they also have, at least potentially, a significant role at: all stages or phases of the rehabilitation process; in all environments of care; across differing foci of intervention; requiring differing levels of skill. These dimensions are captured at the corners of Figure 6.1.

The suggested contents of each box are illustrative rather than definitive. For example, with regard to the stage or phase of rehabilitation we have drawn on the work of Cope and Sundance (1995), but other temporal models would serve equally well. Neither are these dimensions as discrete as Figure 6.1 suggests, and there are areas of inevitable overlap. For example, emergency care will focus predominantly on attaining physiological stability, concentrating interventions at the level of the organ or system, using a range of skills which are likely to be specific or specialist. There are therefore numerous possible combinations inherent in Figure 6.1 but we hope that its dimensions are helpful, in capturing the diversity of the

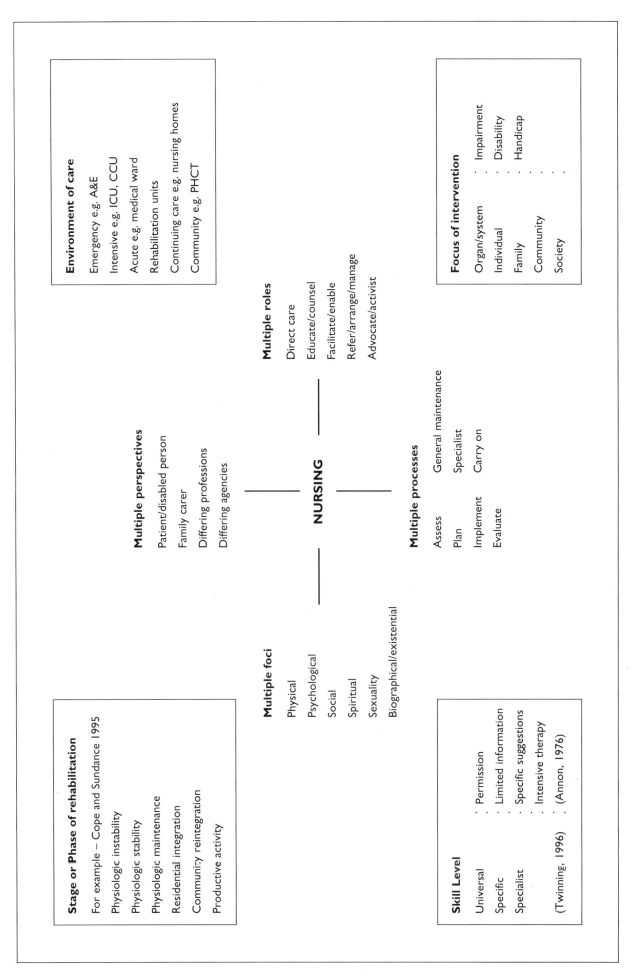

Figure 6.1: Rehabilitation: dimensions of the nursing contribution

The figure contains the following labelled boxes and clusters:

Environment of care

Emergency e.g. A&E
Intensive e.g. ICU, CCU
Acute e.g. medical ward
Rehabilitation units
Continuing care e.g. nursing homes
Community e.g. PHCT

Focus of intervention

Organ/system : Impairment
Individual : Disability
Family : Handicap
Community .
Society .

Multiple perspectives

Patient/disabled person
Family carer
Differing professions
Differing agencies

Multiple roles

Direct care
Educate/counsel
Facilitate/enable
Refer/arrange/manage
Advocate/activist

NURSING

Multiple foci

Physical
Psychological
Social
Spiritual
Sexuality
Biographical/existential

Multiple processes

Assess   General maintenance
Plan   Specialist
Implement   Carry on
Evaluate

Stage or Phase of rehabilitation

For example – Cope and Sundance 1995

Physiologic instability
Physiologic stability
Physiologic maintenance
Residential integration
Community reintegration
Productive activity

Skill Level

Universal : Permission
Specific   : Limited information
Specialist : Specific suggestions
           : Intensive therapy
(Twinning, 1996) : (Annon, 1976)

CHAPTER 6   potential nursing contribution to rehabilitation, and, perhaps more importantly, providing a framework permitting greater specificity in given contexts. It seems to us important that in a particular environment of care that nurses can specify, with some precision: the stage or phase of rehabilitation with which they are concerned; the focus of their interventions; the level of skill required and the knowledge or educational preparation necessary to deliver high quality care.

If the four boxes at the perimeter of Figure 6.1 are designed to help specify the dimensions of the nursing role in a certain context, the centre quadrangle is intended to reflect the multiple roles, processes and foci of nursing interventions and the multiple perspectives to be considered. Again these should be viewed as illustrative rather than exhaustive, but we hope that they are broadly inclusive of the main areas highlighted in the initial review. For example, in addition to providing direct care, the nurse might, in various combinations and circumstances educate or counsel, facilitate or enable, refer, arrange, manage and play an activist role at political or other levels. We feel that the multiple foci are largely self-explanatory, as are most of the multiple processes.

The nurse must be able to assess need in a range of areas and plan, implement and evaluate care. This may well be in the 'traditional areas' such as skin integrity and continence, but the review has also demonstrated enormous potential in a wide range of 'neglected' areas of rehabilitation. Developing the knowledge and skill to intervene in some of these areas seems essential to better rehabilitative care. Such interventions must be evaluated at a more sophisticated level than, for example, that of 'mobilising well'.

On the basis of the initial review, therefore, a framework was produced which outlined the broad dimensions of the nursing role in rehabilitation, as well as deficits in the way rehabilitation is conceptualised and practised. This framework was subjected subsequently to critical scrutiny in the condition-specific reviews to determine if it could be 'recontextualised' to these more disparate areas. It was also necessary to delineate the range of knowledge and skills that nurses require to play a more active role in rehabilitation so as to provide benchmarks for the curriculum analysis. The following chapter considers further the need for a more holistic conceptualisation of rehabilitation, while the subsequent one outlines the type of knowledge and skills that nurses must acquire if they are to play a more integral role.

7.1 Testing the framework

The review of the generic literature identified a number of tensions in current conceptualisations and practice of rehabilitation; these have been reaffirmed recently (Robinson and Batstone, 1996; Baker et al, 1997). Robinson and Batstone (1996) highlight in particular the lack of a shared understanding as to what constitutes rehabilitation, the disadvantages experienced, especially by older users and carers, and the relatively low priority currently afforded to rehabilitation. The potential for greater investment is acknowledged but it is also considered that progress will require a clear conceptual framework mapping the key components and core principles of rehabilitation. Some of their main messages include: rehabilitation is too hospital-dominated; there is little proactive, preventive work; current practice pays little attention to long-term needs; services lack co-ordination; there are communication problems across both professions and agencies.

Robinson and Batstone suggest the present policy initiatives on long-term care and a primary care-led NHS provide a platform on which to build more holistic rehabilitation. However, first consensus must be reached about the parameters of rehabilitation and effort made to *'hear the stories of users and carers'* in order to retain a focus on individual need.

While the present review resulted in an emerging framework with which to consider the potential nursing contribution to rehabilitation, such a role cannot be developed in isolation. Health care in general, and rehabilitation in particular, is an increasingly complex multiprofessional and multiagency undertaking, and, as Robinson and Batstone (1996) suggest, greater consensus and a clearer conceptual framework are needed to begin to *'map'* the parameters of rehabilitation. The five condition-specific reviews undertaken as part of this project were intended to test the adequacy of the framework outlining the nursing contribution and to build a broader conceptualisation of the important elements of rehabilitation itself. As noted earlier, the five conditions were selected to vary along important dimensions of Rolland's model (1988; 1994) – onset, course, outcome and incapacity, thereby providing a more rigorous test for any evolving conceptual framework. Despite the disparate nature of the conditions there was considerable consistency emerging from the themes in the literature, in particular the differences in perception between disabled and chronically ill people and their carers on the one hand, and professionals on the other. As in the initial review, little attention was given to the temporal, biographical and existential elements of rehabilitation, with a finite, physically-orientated model predominating. There was also considerable emphasis on an expanded role for nurses but few concrete suggestions as to how this might be realised. Although there was variation, for example, with more detailed specification of the nursing role in arthritis, the condition-specific reviews were characterised more by similarities than by differences.

A full account of the five separate reviews is not provided here but is available elsewhere if required (Nolan et al, 1997). The intention in the remainder of this report is to identify the commonalties across the reviews, to suggest two contrasting approaches to rehabilitation (the *'restrictive isolated model'* and the *'comprehensive integrative model'*) and to consider the implications of an expanded nurse's role in terms of educational preparation at basic and post-qualifying levels.

7.2 Rehabilitation: contrasting models

One of the most powerful ways of illustrating the limitations of current practice in rehabilitation is to highlight the different perceptions held by disabled and chronically ill people and the professionals who putatively serve them. This theme emerged consistently from each of the condition-specific reviews. This brings into sharp relief the rather empty rhetoric of empowerment and user involvement which is undermined by the inherent power differentials in interactions between health care providers and the recipients of services. Although space precludes a thorough-going discussion at this point a brief consideration of common elements across the conditions reviewed will identify a number of salient points. Those considered here relate specifically to the less tangible and more individual elements of rehabilitation. Literature relating to each of the five conditions reviewed is considered sequentially.

7.2.1 Multiple sclerosis

The temporal, biographical and existential effects of multiple sclerosis (MS) are important and a number of studies have focused on these. Robinson (1989; 1990) described how individuals with MS attempt to make sense of their condition in order to construct a viable life and attain mastery. This involves a number of delicate negotiations which may threaten social relationships, as the individuals and their families engage in a series of multiple dialogues. Robinson (1990) argues that it is therefore imperative that particular attention is given to the personal narratives and life stories of people with MS.

Others similarly talk of the biographical and existential elements of MS in terms of *'meaning'* (Quinn et al, 1995), *'preserving self'* (Fitzgerald and Paterson, 1995) or *'renegotiating life worlds'* and *'interrupted lives'* (Dyck, 1995). The very uncertainty of MS means that expertise is vested largely with the individual rather than the medical system (Price, 1993; Quinn et al, 1995), so it is essential to understand individuals' sources of knowledge. Price (1993) talks of a new paradigm of *'body listening'* whereby MS creates heightened awareness of the body; by listening to their bodies, individuals learn to conserve and maintain energy. Others outline a range of tactics used for this purpose, such as *'pacing'* and changing the physical environment (Quinn et al, 1995), altering routines and household environments, or even moving house (Dyck, 1995).

Quinn et al (1995) describe the temporal unfolding of MS and suggest that adaptation occurs in a number of phases which involve: recognising the disease and its challenges to growth and control; reordering priorities and transforming personal philosophy; acquiring expertise and mastery. Reflecting the gendered nature of the condition, which is more common in women, Dyck (1995) elegantly portrayed the shrinking geographical and personal space women experience, particularly when they leave the workforce. Their lives and experiences become increasingly hidden, as they struggle to *'meet some of the usual expectations associated with women at this time of life'* in terms of contributions to work, family and community. She argues that there is a need to understand the gendered nature of chronic illness and the elements that pertain across gender. Traditional biomedical discourse pay scant attention to such areas.

The need to account for the individualised nature of MS is central to successful interventions, and Quinn et al (1995) suggest that attempts to standardise care *'negate the existential experience'* of those affected. Paradoxically the health service response is to focus on physical elements of care (Kraft et al, 1986; McLaughlin and Zeeberg, 1993) exemplified by the use of *'integrated care pathways'* (Rossiter and Thompson, 1995).

7.2.2 Arthritis

Similar considerations apply in arthritis. From an individual perspective, arthritis, particularly rheumatoid arthritis, impacts on the life course and self-identity. Williams (1984) talks of chronic illness as representing a *'rupture'* in our relationship with the world, and illustrates how people with arthritis strive to make sense of their lives by attempting to realign their biography and reconsider the relationship between self and society. This involves a reconstruction of the past so that the present and future take on a new meaning. Individuals, Williams argues, trace the complex genesis of their condition rather than seeking simple causal explanations. This better reflects the evolution of disability over time (Lambert, 1991). Although arthritis may lack the *'existential gravity'* of more fatal conditions (Williams, 1984) it can have a profoundly disruptive effect requiring individuals to re-establish a sense of personal control. Perry (1991) argues that professionals view disease as a rather abstract concept but that to the individual concerned it is a living reality which leaves them, as Williams and Wood (1988) contend, caught between illness and wellness. These authors describe efforts to maintain reciprocity within relationships, involving a series of negotiations rather than a quest for independence, including negotiation of new roles, adjustment of routines and management of a deviant identity. Independence, in such a context, becomes meaningless, and the interdependence sought involves multiple social and personal compromises. Interventions therefore must focus on the 'concrete reality' of everyday life. Unfortunately, much advice offered by professionals is so marginal to this reality that it is almost impossible to follow (Williams and Wood, 1988).

Similarly, Brown and Williams (1995) contend that until there is a move away from the biomedical model, attempts better to understand an individual perspective will not materialise. They suggest three main themes which relate to individuals' efforts to understand arthritis: helping-seeking behaviour in the face of medical impotence; a search for meaning; and tactics to deal with uncertainty, particularly role incompetence and dependency within family relationships. Others also comment on the difficulties caused by the unpredictable nature of arthritis (Williams, 1984; Ahern et al, 1995).

Professionals, on the other hand, too often seem to be speaking a different language. Williams (1984) posits that the language of science has increasingly rendered it distant from everyday life, a reflection of the abstract view of disease noted by Perry (1991). Even when professionals and patients use the same word it may not have the same meaning (Lambert, 1991). Compounding such potential difficulties Williams and Wood (1988) argue that traditional models of rehabilitation focus on impairment and disability rather than handicap, failing to acknowledge and incorporate the patient's perspective. They describe the emergence of the social model of disability as a reaction against the *'physical self-sufficiency that pervades the rehabilitation literature'* but are critical that the social model itself is *'too atomistic'* and fails fully to account for the multidimensional nature of chronic illness and the delicate *'network of interdependence'* it creates. They call for more creative and flexible options in rehabilitation that might capture the above dynamics more effectively.

Others talk of the need to develop a partnership (Dean-Baar, 1994) which acknowledges that, as Williams (1984) suggests, patients are *'seasoned professionals'* in relation to their condition. This is important in arthritis with its highly individual course (Hosking, 1984), as adaptation is better predicted by subjective perceptions than objective characteristics (Weinberger et al, 1990; Downe-Wamboldt and Melanson, 1995).

7.2.3 Spinal injury

Spinal injury differs significantly from MS and arthritis on important dimensions of Rolland's typology (1988; 1994) especially onset, course and incapacity. Its sudden and traumatic nature gives no time for preparation and the initial insult is usually followed by lengthy hospitalisation. As it affects a generally younger age group, their social support systems are either not well-established or revolve mainly around the parental home. However, following rehabilitation and discharge, spinal injury does not present the same uncertainty or unpredictability as MS and arthritis. Despite such differences however, the literature suggests that many of the challenges are the same, albeit with a differing emphasis.

Spinal injury represents a lifelong challenge, indeed life is usually changed suddenly and irreversibly. This brings into even sharper relief the tensions previously described between the perceptions of health care professionals and the subjective experiences of those with spinal injury. Despite considerable research, adjustment to spinal injury is not well-understood and until fairly recently thinking was dominated by a number of *'stage theories'* (Ragnarsson and Gordon, 1992; Cairns and Baker, 1993; Carpenter, 1994; Spencer et al, 1995), which describe a series of events and stages through which an individual is *expected* to pass, and normally include a phase of depression or dysphoric mood. However, these theories have not been developed from empirical evidence but from professionals' perceptions and experiences (Cairns and Baker, 1993; Carpenter, 1994); there is little empirical support for a normative approach (Ragnarsson and Gordon, 1992; Cairns and Baker, 1993) but such is the influence of these theories that many professionals expect individuals to follow the predicted sequence of adjustment. Somewhat perversely, absence of a depressive mood is often taken as an indication that the patient is adjusting poorly (Dijkers and Cushman, 1990; Whalley-Hammell, 1992; Bodenhamer et al, 1983). The result is a standardised view of a *'typical'* patient (Spencer et al, 1995) based on professional hegemony and expertise. Patients who fail to conform are seen as difficult (Carpenter, 1994). In effect, as Cairns and Baker (1993) note, patients are *'massaged'* to fit a favoured theory, and expected to adapt their behaviour to the views of a dominant group (Carpenter, 1994).

One potentially significant consequence of this is that professionals often have a more pessimistic view of their patient's mood and recovery potential than does the injured person (Dijkers and Cushhan, 1990; Whalley-Hammell, 1992). Formal care providers therefore can significantly under-estimate the life satisfaction of spinal cord injured persons (Whalley-Hammell, 1995) and the fact that such individuals may have a positive outlook has received little attention (Bodenhamer et al, 1983). Oliver et al (1988) termed this dominant view the *'personal tragedy'* model of disability.

Such a standpoint is being increasingly challenged, and there is growing support for an alternative view based on studies of the experience of people with spinal injury. Much of this literature describes themes strikingly similar to those developed in MS and arthritis concerning the biographical and existential elements of illness and injury.

Dewis (1989), in a study of adolescents adjusting to spinal injury, argues that care providers (particularly nurses) must seek to understand the *'meanings'* affected individuals accord to events. Their prime concern is to *'carve out'* a new identity based on feelings of self-worth and value, and they become skilled in presenting themselves as *'normal'*, often in ingenious ways, usually without the help of formal care providers.

Yoshida (1993; 1994) also views the reconstruction of self as essential but considers that there are two *'selves'* (the non-disabled and the disabled self), each struggling to achieve a balance. The non-disabled self still exists but has to reconcile itself with the disabled self. This, according to Yoshida, necessitates a *'pendular'* reconstruction involving *'identity transformation'*. This is a dynamic process represented diagrammatically in Figure 7.1.

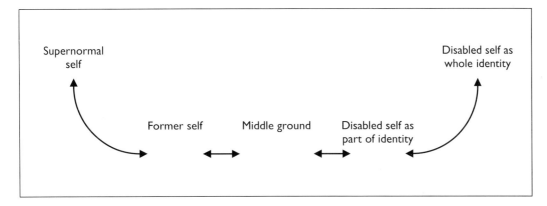

Figure 7.1: The process of identity transformation
(after Yoshida, 1994)

The middle ground represents the most satisfactory outcome where 'core' attributes of the former self are retained but integrated with the disabled self so that a new identity emerges. Unfortunately, rehabilitation focuses almost exclusively on the disabled self, preoccupied as it is with physical recovery. This, Yoshida (1994) argues, leads to neglect of the non-disabled self with three largely negative, consequences:

- lack of preparation for living a 'normal' life

- lack of attention to sexual concerns

- failure to individualise programmes of rehabilitation.

Carpenter (1994) also outlines the *'disability experience'* in spinal cord injury, describing the quest to rediscover self, redefine disabilities and establish a new identity. This is a longitudinal process, yet rehabilitation increasingly focuses on acute physical care, failing to pay attention to the nature of the individual pre-injury (Spoltore and O'Brien, 1995; Spencer et al, 1995).

7.2.4   Myocardial infarction

In contrast to the other conditions in this review, there is a dearth of qualitative research on cardiac rehabilitation. This may explain why, despite extensive research, the adjustment process following myocardial infarction (MI) is poorly understood (Johnson, 1991; Thompson et al, 1995). Nevertheless, the limited literature available recognises that professional perspectives may differ from those of patients (Johnson and Morse, 1990) and that the goals of rehabilitation should be meaningful to patients (Malan, 1992).

The few studies that have adopted a qualitative and temporal approach reach conclusions remarkably similar to those pertaining to MS, arthritis and spinal cord injury. Hawthorne (1991) stresses the importance of adopting a temporal dimension and advocated the use of the trajectory model (Corbin and Strauss, 1988; 1991). A temporal perspective is also highlighted by Ford (1989), who suggests that two years after MI men have relearned to *'listen to their bodies'*, a process described earlier relating to MS. Ford (1989) suggests that this might help explain non-compliance with treatment. It is therefore important that professionals appreciate how individuals perceive the past and the present when considering a potential future.

The most detailed qualitative study describing adjustment to MI is that of Johnson (Johnson and Morse, 1990; Johnson, 1991), which presents a model of the adjustment process comprising four phases, the main aim of each being to retain or regain control. These stages are seen as iterative and recursive rather than linear, often following a cyclical pattern. The four stages, each with a number of sub-processes are:

- defending the self

- coming to terms

- learning to live

- living again.

'*Defending the self*' involves attempts to normalise or trivialise the initial symptoms of MI in order to deny the potential seriousness of events. However, once help is sought patients tend to distance themselves from their circumstances and enter a period of unreality. '*Coming to terms*' involves facing one's own mortality and making sense of the infarction. Subsequently, in order for progress to be made, it is necessary to face limitations and look to the future. Johnson (1991) contrasts the perceptions that differentiate a positive attitude from a '*wait and see*' philosophy (Table 7.1).

Positive attitude	'Wait and see'
Confidence in recovery	Fear of disability
'Knowing' the cause	Anger/confusion
Grateful for a second chance	Why me?
Specific rehabilitation plans	Fear/uncertainty
Limitations seen as manageable	Limitations insurmountable

Table 7.1: Effects of attitude on coming to terms with illness and disability
(adapted from Johnson, 1991)

Subsequently, '*learning to live*' is a process of preserving self, minimising uncertainty, and developing new '*guidelines*' for living. It is important that individuals have a sense of progress and, according to Johnson (1991), they often look to professionals for reassurance that they are '*doing well*'. Johnson (1991) suggests a four-cell matrix highlighting the importance of congruence between individual and professional perceptions of positive progress.

In order to '*live again*' individuals must accept their limitations, focus on the positive aspects of their situation, and attain a sense of mastery. Those who fail to achieve this balance '*abandon the struggle*', seeing their situation as hopeless and insurmountable. The authors acknowledge the need to develop and refine their model, but it is consistent with much of the psychological literature on adjustment to MI, which stresses the importance of correcting erroneous misconceptions and facilitating a sense of hope and control (Lewin, 1995).

Taking a different focus and timescale, Thompson et al (1995) examined the first month post infarction, for both sufferer and partner. They highlight the dearth of information and advice received, particularly by the partner, and describe how emotional reactions such as fear of another attack can lead to over-protection. These authors believe there is a lack of attention to the needs of both sufferer and partner in the month following discharge, and advocate the development of '*novel*' services, such as systems of monitoring and support by community nurses, coronary care teams or drop-in centres. They also present a case for more qualitative in-depth studies on the effects of MI.

7.2.5　Stroke

As with MI there is relatively little detailed qualitative work on the consequences of stroke. Doolittle (1988) argues that our knowledge of stroke survivors' adaptation over time is sparse and although she and others (Doolittle, 1991; 1992; 1994; Häggström et al, 1994; Lewinter and Mikkelsen, 1995a; 1995b) have attempted to redress the balance, these accounts are not as well-developed or as sophisticated as the biographical, existential and temporal models highlighted in other parts of this review. However, accounts that are available are consistent with the literature relating to MS, arthritis, spinal injury and MI, talking of the need to find a new identity, to reorder a disordered body and to renegotiate social relationships (Lewinter and Mikkelsen, 1995a). Doolittle (1994) charts the recovery of the social body and the work needed to recapture *'bodily knowledge'*. Using the metaphor of *'life as a tapestry'*, Häggström et al (1994) identify four main themes in stroke recovery:

- uncertainty

- sadness and meaning

- gratification, hope and satisfaction

- isolation.

The relative balance between these themes reflects the potential for stroke to result in *'long-term misery'* (Young and Gladman, 1995).

Although not adopting a qualitative methodology, Glass and Maddox (1992) argue that stroke recovery should be conceptualised as a *'psychosocial transition'*, which challenges the assumptive worlds of those affected, requiring new definitions of self and a renegotiation of roles within established relationships.

What emerges most forcibly from these, and related studies is: the importance of focusing on the values, goals, aspirations and meanings of stroke survivors themselves (Chiou and Burnett, 1985; Doolittle, 1991; 1992; 1994; Folden, 1994; Boynton de Sepulveda and Chang, 1994; Pound et al, 1995; Lewinter and Mikkelsen, 1995a). Consequently Doolittle (1991) notes that emphasis should be placed on the impact of stroke on the person's life rather than simply the extent of neurological damage.

The above focus on the differences in perception between chronically ill and disabled people and rehabilitation professionals across all five conditions reviewed has highlighted the consistency between literature from disparate sources and differing conditions. This was not the only area in which themes emerged from the condition-specific reviews which transcended the nature of the disease, suggesting a consensus in the literature (see Nolan et al (1997) for full discussion). These themes are summarised in Table 7.2 which illustrates a number of deficits in current rehabilitation practice. These conclusions reinforce Oliver's (1993) contention that *'all is not well in the kingdom of rehabilitation'* and highlight the need for a radical rethink of the aims, purposes and organisation of services.

As Robinson and Batstone (1996) argue, an element of consensus is required if there is to be an informed debate, but such a consensus is hampered by the absence of an agreed definition of rehabilitation. These authors argue that rehabilitation must be distinguished from acute care and continuing care and be viewed as a distinct stage in health care delivery, but we would not fully agree. Whilst subscribing to the need for a clear framework and acknowledging the fundamental differences between a curative orientation and other, more diffuse, health care needs, we believe that the distinction between rehabilitation and continuing or long-term care is increasingly spurious and indeed the source of many of the tensions identified in the review.

Such a differentiation might be administratively convenient, but it has little meaning to disabled and chronically ill people and their families. Rather it makes a mockery of the trite sentiments underpinning the rhetoric of 'seamless care' and fragments the experience of a daily life often involving continued contact with the health and social care services. It is time, Robinson and Batstone (1996) advise, to hear the stories of users and carers, whose voices have been muted for too long; they see the *'head of steam'* currently fuelling debates about rehabilitation as providing the necessary impetus. We would wholly endorse this sentiment, and to stimulate further debate, suggest that rehabilitation can be conceptualised in terms of two overarching models – the *'restricted isolated model'* and the *'comprehensive integrative model'*, the characteristics of which are illustrated in Figure 7.2.

We see these models as ideal types, serving an heuristic function, rather than being literal representations. Each comprises multiple continua, the poles of which are depicted in Figure 7.2. There are therefore numerous potential variations both within and between continua, making an infinite number of combinations. While a truly comprehensive model may indeed be ideal, and therefore unobtainable, we hope these models will serve their purpose in stimulating debate and believe that the further rehabilitation practice moves towards the comprehensive end of the spectrum on each criterion the more it will resonate with the stories of users and carers.

We believe that the development of a more comprehensive and integrative approach to rehabilitation will not be achieved until greater attention is paid to the deficits in practice summarised in Table 7.2. This will mean adopting a constructively critical approach which pays more than passing attention to patients and their carers. Furthermore, concerted action is needed if the rhetoric of interdisciplinary teamwork is to be translated into a workable system of care delivery. The nursing profession has a potentially important role to play, particularly if the neglected aspects of the nursing contribution outlined in Figure 6.1 are developed further. This has a number of implications for the education and training of practitioners at both qualifying and post-qualifying levels, which are considered in the penultimate chapter.

- Imbalance between professional perspectives and those of disabled people, particularly the emphasis placed on the physical outcomes of rehabilitation to the neglect of existential and biographical perspectives important to disabled and chronically ill people

- A failure to individualise rehabilitation programmes

- Insufficient information, advice and education

- Insufficient attention to emotional needs

- Insufficient attention to psychological needs

- Insufficient attention to work, vocational aspects

- Insufficient attention to specific areas such as sexuality

- Failure to address the temporal aspects of rehabilitation such as transitions through the health care system, lack of co-ordination and fragmented services, insufficient/absent long-term follow-up

- Neglect of issues surrounding gender, culture, ethnicity and so on

- Neglect of the needs of family carers

- Insufficient attention to the attitudinal and environmental barriers to the full integration of disabled and chronically ill people into society

Table 7.2: Areas of deficit in current rehabilitation practice

---

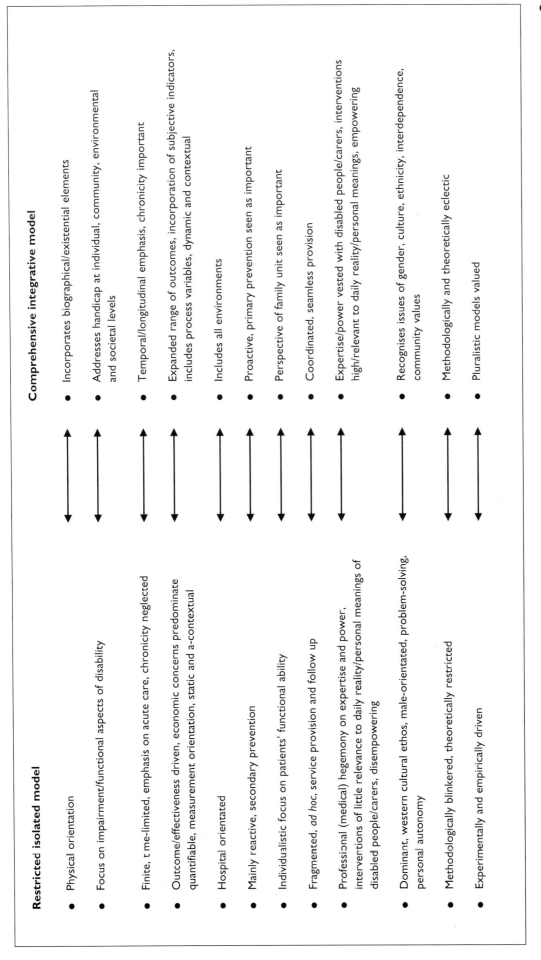

Restricted isolated model

- Physical orientation

- Focus on impairment/functional aspects of disability

- Finite, time-limited, emphasis on acute care, chronicity neglected

- Outcome/effectiveness driven, economic concerns predominate quantifiable, measurement orientation, static and a-contextual

- Hospital orientated

- Mainly reactive, secondary prevention

- Individualistic focus on patients' functional ability

- Fragmented, *ad hoc*, service provision and follow up

- Professional (medical) hegemony on expertise and power, interventions of little relevance to daily reality/personal meanings of disabled people/carers, disempowering

- Dominant, western cultural ethos, male-orientated, problem-solving, personal autonomy

- Methodologically blinkered, theoretically restricted

- Experimentally and empirically driven

Comprehensive integrative model

- Incorporates biographical/existential elements

- Addresses handicap at individual, community, environmental and societal levels

- Temporal/longitudinal emphasis, chronicity important

- Expanded range of outcomes, incorporation of subjective indicators, includes process variables, dynamic and contextual

- Includes all environments

- Proactive, primary prevention seen as important

- Perspective of family unit seen as important

- Coordinated, seamless provision

- Expertise/power vested with disabled people/carers, interventions high/relevant to daily reality/personal meanings, empowering

- Recognises issues of gender, culture, ethnicity, interdependence, community values

- Methodologically and theoretically eclectic

- Pluralistic models valued

Figure 7.2: Rehabilitation: contrasting models

PREPARING FOR A MORE ACTIVE ROLE

8.1 Knowledge and skills for practice

The literature on the nurse's contribution to rehabilitation suggests that while current roles are poorly developed there is considerable potential for nurses to play a greater part in a number of areas, summarised in Table 6.1 and Figure 6.1. The condition-specific reviews largely reinforced these conclusions with similar roles being identified across the five areas of rehabilitation, albeit with slightly varying emphasis.

In order to fulfil these roles adequately an extensive knowledge and skill base is required. An illustrative list of some of the of roles and an indicative knowledge base are summarised in Table 8.1. However, despite it being constantly reiterated that nurses are ideally placed to fulfil a varied range of roles most of these are in areas where there are the greatest deficits in current practice. It seems therefore that there is room for considerable improvement in rehabilitation generally and the nursing contribution in particular. This is exemplified by the situation in stroke rehabilitation which represents a paradigm case capturing many of the current tensions and dilemmas in the rehabilitation literature.

Myco (1984) argues that although lip service is paid to the nursing role in stroke rehabilitation, the role is ill-defined. She believes nurses must take prime responsibility for this situation as they have failed to specify their involvement; consequently, they might build on or maintain care provided by other disciplines, but are not expected to initiate action. More recently, Wild (1994) questions whether stroke rehabilitation is a productive use of nursing time or is more appropriately the domain of the therapy disciplines, and argues that nurses are unable to articulate clearly what they do, let alone evaluate its effectiveness.

The question, she contends, is whether nurses should be *'innovative practitioners'* or simply *'direct doers'*. Nurses' potential role in stroke rehabilitation is graphically captured by Anderson:

> *'Nurses appear to be the key figures influencing the quality of the patient's stay in hospital. It is likely that more comforting, counselling and communication are provided to stroke patients by nursing staff than by any other group in the hospital, they spend more time with patients than any other group, and may be most knowledgeable about problems ... Altogether, nurses appear to be the most critical elements in the patient's experience of daily life in hospital ... The balance between expressions of interest and indifference may have a profound effect on the patient's attitude to stroke and to themselves.'* (Anderson, 1992 p62-63)

However, the nurse's role in stroke rehabilitation remains *'vague and ill-defined'* (Gibbon, 1991; Irwin, 1996) and evaluation is often confined to such limited observations as *'sitting in the chair'* (Wild, 1994). If nurses are to realise their potential role they must acquire the range of knowledge and skills outlined in Table 8.1. This will necessitate considerable reorientation of educational preparation at basic and post-qualifying levels, as the analyses of course curricula undertaken in this project revealed. There was limited attention to chronic illness, disability and rehabilitation in a range of diploma and degree common foundation and adult branch programmes, community nursing and specialist courses for those working with older people (for a fuller account, see Nolan et al, 1997).

Role	Knowledge/skills
Assessment of physical condition, delivery of skilled care, prevention of secondary complications	• Detailed physiology and related anatomy and pathology of relevant conditions e.g. stroke, MS etc. • Knowledge of normal physiology and a range of therapeutic interventions • Knowledge of a range of measurement indices and their operational bases
Education/counselling	• Detailed knowledge of adult learning and counselling theory, group facilitation processes etc. • Ability to assess readiness, capacity and motivation to learn. Assessment of preferred learning style
Psychosocial interventions	• Ability to assess mood and psychological state • Understanding of a range of theoretical areas, particularly stress theory • Ability to assess appropriateness of coping styles and modify accordingly. Use of cognitive-behavioural models
Family carers	• Detailed knowledge of family systems theories • Ability to assess family dynamics
Sexuality	• Ability to address sexuality on an individual basis • Knowledge and skill in counselling and intervention techniques relevant to identified need
Co-ordinating role, liaison and facilitating transitions through the health care system	• Detailed knowledge of multidisciplinary working • High level of communication skills, diplomacy, assertiveness • Knowledge of service delivery systems

Table 8.1: Indicative areas of knowledge and skills necessary for fulfilling a variety of potential nursing roles in rehabilitation

8.2   Specific model or eclectic knowledge base?

Furthermore, nurses need not only awareness of theoretical principles underpinning care but must be able to translate such knowledge into skilled interventions. One way that the nursing role in rehabilitation can become more apparent is by using an overreaching theory or model (Gale and Gaylard, 1996; Waters, 1996). Some advocate the use of existing nursing models such as Orem (Waters, 1987; Gale and Gaylard, 1996) or Roper, Logan and Tierney (Gale and Gaylard, 1996), although there is increasing recognition of the need for *'an accepted nursing rehabilitation model'* (Waters, 1996).

A number of potential candidates exist in the literature, for example the Corbin and Strauss (1992) model recommended by Woog (1992), based on the trajectory framework described earlier. This model has the advantage of having been developed from the experiences of chronically ill and disabled people and adapted and tested in a nursing context (Woog, 1992). The model suggests a number of nursing interventions, including, direct care, teaching, counselling, referring, arranging and monitoring. However, central to the model is placing prime responsibility with disabled people and their families, with nursing activities complementing and augmenting their efforts. In applying the model to nursing interventions, Corbin and Strauss (1992) suggest an approach similar to the nursing process (Table 8.2) and outline a number of factors that may influence the management of chronic illness and disability, summarised in Table 8.3. In addition to the model of Corbin and Strauss (1992), frameworks such as the *'illness-constellation model'* (Morse and Johnson, 1991) also require further empirical scrutiny.

Although not falling into the category of a specific model or framework other generalised approaches such as the stress/coping paradigm appear frequently in the literature. Greater specificity is required so that these concepts can be applied by *nurses in a rehabilitative context*. Hymovich and Hagopian (1992) provide just such a framework in their *'contingency model of long-term care'*, which synthesises many elements described in this review and identifies how they may be utilised by nurses. The contingency model deliberately incorporates elements from diverse disciplines (psychology, sociology, nursing, management, education and others), recognising that such varied sources of knowledge are essential if the needs of chronically ill and disabled people and their families are to be met. Underpinning the model are a number of assumptions which reflect many of the points raised in this review:

- subjective perceptions are essential to an understanding of how people act

- there are both unique and common responses to chronic illness

- all members of the family need to be included

- the needs of chronically ill and disabled people and their families are complex and require a team approach

- disabled people and their families are an integral part of the health care team

- it is possible to influence a person's internal motivation.

Step 1. Determine the client's and family's response to and their present management of the illness using:
- illness
- biography
- everyday activities

Establish goals of intervention

Step 2. Assess conditions influencing management (see Table 8.3)

Step 3. Define and refine the focus of the intervention using steps 1 and 2

Step 4. Provide interventions which may include:
- direct care
- teaching
- counselling
- referring
- arranging
- monitoring

Step 5. Evaluate effectiveness of the intervention – this requires a long-term perspective accounting for factors identified in steps 1 and 2

Table 8.2: Applying the trajectory framework to nursing
(adapted from Corbin and Strauss, 1992)

- Type/amount/complexity/duration of technology and treatment
- Resources available, both human and financial
- Patient's experience of the illness
- Motivation of patient and family
- Setting of care
- Lifestyle and beliefs
- Interactions and relationships between participants in care
- Type and stage of illness
- Symptoms
- Political and economic factors

Table 8.3: Factors influencing the management of chronic illness
(adapted from Corbin and Strauss, 1992)

The model is essentially systems-driven, based primarily on the family unit; it comprises five distinct but interacting and overlapping areas, hence the term 'contingency':

- systems: individual, family, community and society

- time: past, present and future

- contingency variables: orientation to life (values/attitudes/beliefs)

    stressors

    coping strategies, strengths and needs

- level of functioning: developmental and situational

- nursing care.

The model identifies a number of areas for nursing intervention, but the authors highlight the importance of team-working and collaboration, placing the disabled person and family at the centre of the team. Hymovich and Hagopian (1992) point out that their framework is still evolving and that further research is needed to provide more complete answers to many of the questions it raises. Nevertheless, it appears flexible enough to incorporate new knowledge as it emerges and, although presented as a way of organising nursing interventions, lends itself to multidisciplinary application, suggesting that the contingency model merits more widespread development.

Another area where further developments are required is the role of family carers. Nolan et al (1996) advocate the use of a broadly interpreted stress-coping model with carers and outline a number of general principles which should underpin practice:

- identify and reinforce carers' appropriate coping responses

- identify and seek to reduce inappropriate coping responses

- help carers to develop new coping resources and responses

- augment existing coping resources by building larger support networks

- services should substitute for carers only when the above interventions prove unsuccessful

- services should not support carers beyond the point where their own health suffers

- services must adopt a more enabling, facilitative role, working with carers as partners in a way which is sensitive to their expertise and stage of caring history.

Such models also merit further exploration as a framework for use with both disabled people and their carers in rehabilitation. However, if they are to prove useful Nolan et al (1996) argue that mechanisms must be in place to facilitate their practical application, and present a range of indices to 'assess' the difficulties carers face, the satisfactions they employ and the coping efforts they utilise (Nolan and Grant, 1992a; Nolan et al, 1995). The indices are not intended to be applied in a deterministic fashion, to compare carers in a normative way with others, but to produce an *individual profile* of each carer's circumstances, providing the basis not only for assessment but also for designing appropriate interventions and their subsequent evaluation.

Recently the rehabilitation literature has recognised the validity of measures producing an individual profile as in instruments such as the Rehabilitation Activities Profile (Laman and Lankhorst, 1994; Van Bennekom et al, 1995; Lankhorst et al, 1995), a principle also acknowledged by others (Raeburn and Rootman, 1996). This raises other debates about the value of methodological approaches such as the randomised controlled trial, and the use of single case experimental models is increasingly advocated (Ottenbacher, 1990; Brummel-Smith, 1993; Pollock et al, 1993; Ward and McIntosh, 1993).

Issues such as these are increasingly relevant for nurses, many of whom eschew a measurement-orientated approach. However, a resource-constrained health service requires *some* indication of success, so it is encouraging that nurses are advancing more patient-centred approaches to measurement, for example, of physical ability in rehabilitation (Grenville and Lyne, 1995). The dearth of good theory underpinning many existing measures was discussed in Section 3.1, and Trexler and Fordyce (1996) note that such difficulties are compounded by the fact that most practitioners accept measures uncritically, unaware of the principles on which they are founded. The ability to critique existing measures and suggest or develop more appropriate instruments appears to be an essential skill for nurses in rehabilitation, particularly at specialist and advanced levels, and needs to be reflected in their educational preparation.

Utilising more specific constructs such as powerlessness (Miller, 1992b), hope and hopelessness (Farran et al, 1995) or quality of life (Renwick et al, 1996) other authors provide a conceptual basis for rehabilitative care which could help to inform current practice. A number of mid-range theories have been referred to in this review, for example, those of Morse and O'Brien (1995), Thorne (1993) or Nolan et al (1996). Although many were developed only recently, others have been available for some time, and it is disappointing that they have not been utilised and refined within a rehabilitation context.

At a more specific level the frameworks for addressing difficult areas such as guilt (Flannery, 1990) and sexuality (Rieve, 1989) already described are useful. The staged approach to sexuality advocated by Rieve (1989) seems particularly helpful and could be expanded and applied to rehabilitative nursing in general to assist in the identification of various levels of practice. For example, the model's first two levels – creating a climate in which issues such as sexuality and guilt can be discussed, and providing limited information – seem legitimate skills for *any* qualified nurse. The use of 'specific suggestions' relating to a given issue may be the remit of the specialist practitioner whereas 'intensive therapy' is more appropriate for advanced practice or specialist disciplines (clinical psychology, sexual counsellors and so on). Such a framework could also be applied to the range of psychological and psychotherapeutic interventions described by authors such as Twinning (1996) and Knight (1996) to determine which, if any, could be within the practice repertoire of all qualified nurses in rehabilitation settings and which confined to specialist and advanced practitioners.

On the basis of the above it seems reasonable to argue that nursing, just as Barnard (1995) suggests of the concept of hope, is a *'boundary discipline'*, that does not belong to a specific intellectual or theoretical tradition but draws on a range of knowledge emanating from disparate sources. Such debates are manifest in the wider nursing literature and highlight tensions between the need for a unique body of nursing knowledge or the carefully considered application and refinement of a more varied knowledge base to nursing practice. Both the general and nursing specific literature on rehabilitation place considerable emphasis on the latter approach, advocating the need to draw upon a wide range of sources of knowledge (Gerhardt, 1989; Friedland and McColl, 1992; Preston, 1994; Thorne, 1993; RCN, 1994; Hoeman, 1996). Table 8.1 indicates just how extensive this knowledge base might be.

However, there is a need for caution when considering such all-embracing lists. While rehabilitation nurses may be introduced to all these sources of knowledge, the risk remains that it will be at such a level of generality, superficiality or both that they cannot meaningfully apply knowledge in a given context. It also begs the question as to how such an extensive theoretical content can be covered within the confines of a given programme of education and *who* is capable of teaching it. The provision of general principles is laudable and necessary in setting a context and framework, but the transformation of such information into practically useful knowledge (Paul and Heaslip, 1995) also needs to be addressed. Having advocated the need for a broader conceptualisation of the nurse's role in rehabilitation, paradoxically there must also be a complementary element of greater specificity. Moreover, nurses cannot operate in isolation and their programmes of preparation must to prepare them for a more extensive role in the multidisciplinary team.

The central importance of teamwork to rehabilitation raises significant tensions for nurse education. The first is that concepts of teamwork have to be explored in detail during training and explicit attention given to how teamwork can be incorporated into practice. This requires consideration not only of the underlying theoretical principles but also of how these can be translated into a workable reality. As Barnes (1993) notes, simply bringing people together in the vague hope that they will work effectively is not sufficient. Preparation for team-working must therefore figure more prominently in training (Diller, 1990; Wood, 1993); it should include *'field-based experiences'* (McCormick and Goldman, 1979) and equip staff with sufficient knowledge of psychology to help them recognise and deal with the emotions and conflict teamwork can generate (Trexler and Fordyce, 1996). As a basic minimum, therefore, nurses need a *thorough* understanding of the philosophy and values underpinning the practice of related health care disciplines, including medicine and the paramedical professions. This should be included in basic preparation and reinforced at post-qualification levels. This is unlikely to be achieved by a few token hours input on the role of physiotherapy or occupational therapy, but requires a systematic comparison which seeks to render explicit the implicit assumptions underpinning other professions and their practice.

Some form of shared learning represents the ideal scenario and this has been reinforced in the recent White Paper on the future of the NHS (Secretary of State, 1996a) and the report of the Standing Medical and Nursing and Midwifery Advisory Committee (SNMAC, 1996), which states *'The lack of early interdisciplinary training helps to perpetuate misunderstandings about different professional approaches and their underlying values'*. A consideration of how this deficit might be addressed within basic nurse education is required if there is to be a general improvement in team-working. It is *essential* if the changes in rehabilitation practice envisaged here are to occur. The ultimate solution may be to work towards the sort of generic transdisciplinary professional suggested by Hollingbery (1994); this is unrealistic in the foreseeable future, but some form of greater understanding of professional roles must be engendered.

The purpose of this review was to identify the nurse's current role in rehabilitation, to consider how it might develop and to identify the implications for nurse education and training. It was also envisaged that a framework might emerge to aid conceptual development and practice innovation. Rehabilitation is still evolving and likely to continue to do so and what is most useful in such circumstances is not an all-embracing model to direct practice but rather a framework within which to cast rehabilitation so that a range of options can be identified. The literature indicates that numerous options exist, emanating from disparate theoretical perspectives. Many are sufficiently focused to be of practical relevance, but others require further empirical testing and refinement. Nursing needs to identify these sources of knowledge and harness them to improve care and practice in rehabilitation.

It is hoped that the parameters of a legitimate nursing role in rehabilitation within the context of the multi (inter) disciplinary team have been elucidated and that this will assist both the development of roles and specific interventions. It would be inappropriate for this review to suggest which interventions might be most useful, as this requires further empirical work and conceptual refinement. It is apparent, however, that techniques which more closely align professional practice with the needs of chronically ill and disabled people and their carers are essential if rehabilitation practice is to advance. We have termed such an approach a *comprehensive integrative model.* Nurses can provide the bridgehead towards such a more holistic orientation but must be adequately prepared for the required changes in practice. The concluding chapter outlines a number of implications for the development of practice in rehabilitation.

'Nurses are in an unique; ideal; key; pivotal position to ...'

'The role of the nurse in stroke patient rehabilitation ... lacks any framework for rehabilitative rationale essential to continuity of care.'
(Myco, 1984 p434)

'It is extremely difficult to have any meaningful discussions about rehabilitation when it means so many different things to different people.'
(Robinson and Batstone, 1996 p23)

9.1   The nursing role

Henderson's (1980) assertion that nurses are *'rehabilitators par excellence'* is probably one of the most frequent 'sound bites' appearing in the nursing literature on rehabilitation and this is reflected in the above composite quote which we have constructed from several sources which suggest the poll position that the profession putatively holds in rehabilitative care. Some years ago Myco (1984) questioned the basis of Henderson's confidence, arguing that the nursing contribution to rehabilitation was something of a chimera, a point since reiterated a number of times (Gibbon, 1991; O'Connor, 1993; Wild, 1994). These latter authors contend that the nursing role lacks clarity and that a well-researched, solidly defensible set of interventions is not apparent. Alluding to stroke rehabilitation, O'Connor (1993) argues that nurses increasingly fulfil a *'non-therapeutic managerial role or a non-specific under-study role'* and that there are no unique rehabilitative interventions that can be called 'nursing'.

Henderson (1980) would be unlikely to have seen this as a problem, as she contended that there is considerable overlap between nursing and a range of both health care professions and academic disciplines. To her the 'uniqueness' of nursing was the provision of humanistic, *'basic nursing care'* on a 24-hour, seven-day-a-week basis. She viewed modern health care as impersonal and contended that one of the main nursing skills is to *'get under the patient's skin'* in order to deliver *'humanistic and psychosocial aspects of care as well as the technical skills'*. Although Henderson did not elaborate upon her vision of rehabilitation, she was concerned to preserve the *'essence of nursing in a technological age'*. Her thoughts were in many ways prophetic as her paper preceded the proliferation of debates about a specialist or extended nursing role and in this context her arguments are equally relevant nearly 20 years later.

She fully acknowledged the importance of nurses working closely with medical and other colleagues, highlighting the resultant and inevitable overlap of roles, and admonished nurses, doctors and other health care workers *'to continuously assess the role or function of every category of worker'* so that patients would not suffer as a consequence of boundary disputes. She foresaw the present emphasis on evidence-based care and urged nurses to take a full and active part in elucidating their practice, abandoning the *'cookbook'* mentality that she considered pervasive in nurse education.

Underpinning her position however was the desire to develop the humanistic aspects of nursing. She believed this required a radical change in the focus and orientation of health care towards sections of society who were *'conspicuously neglected'*, such as the *'chronically ill, the mentally retarded, the prison population and the institutionalised aged'*, arguing that it was such groups who would most benefit from *'expert humanistic nursing'*.

Henderson's (1980) conclusions mirror those of this review which has identified a number of tensions and contradictions in current rehabilitation, not least of which is the present emphasis on the technical (acute, finite, outcome driven) at the expense of the humanistic (temporal, biographical, existential). It therefore seems appropriate to paraphrase Henderson's thesis and to consider how to preserve the essence of rehabilitation in a technological age.

9.2 What is rehabilitation?

Oliver (1993) poses the rhetorical question *'What's so wonderful about walking?'* to highlight one of the fundamental iniquities in the way rehabilitation is currently conceptualised: the imposition of the standards of the able-bodied as the benchmark of a successful outcome. For those of us able to walk the question seems naïve, of course walking is wonderful. On the other hand for someone who can no longer walk and will never do so again, the question is highly relevant. To constantly strive for that which is unobtainable is to court continual failure and, according to Finkelstein (1981), results in *'... endless soul-destroying hours trying to approximate to able-bodied standards'*. In critiquing existing rehabilitation practice Oliver (1993) does not advocate that the baby be thrown out with the bath water but argues that some issues surrounding rehabilitation have barely been considered. Foremost among these is the emphasis on 'physicality' and the underlying ideology and power differentials that this subsumes.

By highlighting the importance of the existential, biographical and temporal dimensions of rehabilitation and arguing that the rehabilitative process should include primary prevention as well as secondary and tertiary interventions, this review endorses many of Oliver's arguments (1993). Rehabilitation should not be limited to the restoration of function, no matter how inclusive the definition of function that is employed. It also needs to extend beyond the disabled person, to include the family, community, society and environment. As with Oliver's position this is not to say that physical functioning is unimportant but rather that there is far more to it than this.

9.3 Opportunities and barriers

In considering the current nursing role in rehabilitation we suggest that there is a need for both generic and specialist functions. However, both roles are at present under-developed, constrained by the failure of most nurses to recognise rehabilitation as an important component of their practice and compounded by the limited attention to rehabilitation, disability and chronic illness in education and training. Despite this, there exists considerable potential for nurses to take the lead in forging new directions in rehabilitation practice and address many of the current limitations. However, this will mean recognising both the opportunities presented and the barriers to be overcome.

Earlier, Symington's (1994) seven 'megatrends' were used to set this review in context and they are utilised again here in order to highlight the opportunities and barriers to rehabilitation generally and the nurse's role in particular.

9.3.1 Demographics

The first factor considered by Symington is the changing demography of illness and disability, particularly the rise in chronic illnesses and increasing numbers of older people. This theme recurred throughout the review and there is now a more widespread appreciation that chronic illness represents the greatest challenge to modern health services. It is equally clear that such conditions are the least well-catered for, primarily due to the continued application of an acute simple disease model rather than a chronic complex illness model (Pawlson, 1994), or as we suggest a *restricted isolated* approach rather than a *comprehensive integrative* one. We urge the need for caution if we are to avoid current efforts to develop specialist and advanced nursing roles exacerbating this situation.

It seems to us that the more nurses take on roles once associated with junior doctors the less likely is the profession to address important areas in chronicity and rehabilitation. In order to develop a balanced perspective, nurses need a more complete understanding of the nature and diversity of chronic diseases and disability and the temporal nature and multiple impacts of such conditions. Many nursing authors cited in this review believe that chronicity is a concept at the heart of nursing and yet a consideration of this was virtually absent from the curricula reviewed, even those concerned with the needs of older people (see Nolan et al, 1997 for a full account). Useful frameworks, for example, the ICIDH, were rarely referred to explicitly and topics such as the needs of disabled people during periods of hospitalisation were similarly absent, despite the fact that deficits in current practice are often attributed to nurses. There is a clear need for more research in this area and it must be considered whether chronicity in general and a number of more specific models and theories receive sufficient explicit attention in the curricula of programmes of preparation at both pre- and post-registration levels. This is particularly important in view of the prevailing demographic trends and the rise in both the absolute number and proportion of frail older people. There is a lack of an adequate theoretical basis for health care in advanced old age and this is an area to which nursing could make a significant contribution. This is unlikely to be realised if the discourse of independence and problem-solving remains in the ascendancy.

9.3.2 Emancipation and integration of disabled people

The second area highlighted by Symington is the emancipation of disabled people and this might usefully be considered together with the third 'megatrend', moves towards the integration of disabled people into society. Authors advocating a social model of disability would probably stand askance at Symington's suggestions, asking for evidence to support such emancipation and integration, arguing that a disabling society is still manifest. It would be hard to disagree with such a position; while the language of empowerment, facilitation and partnership pervades the policy rhetoric and the professional literature, the accounts of service users, particularly chronically ill and disabled people, stand as an indictment of the failure to deliver on such promises.

As this review has demonstrated, there now exists a considerable literature highlighting the importance of establishing a relationship of trust with disabled people and paying due regard to the existential and biographical aspects of their lives. Numerous models and mid-range theories can be drawn upon to inform this aspect of care, many developed specifically by, or for, nurses. Furthermore the notion of partnership extends beyond disabled people to include their families. There is also a substantial literature on family systems and other models of intervention which might usefully be incorporated into mainstream nurse education. Moreover, attention to external factors such as the built environment, together with genuine efforts to construe chronically ill people as healthy must also be reflected, with varying degrees of sophistication, at both qualifying and post-qualifying levels. The literature suggests that these topics currently receive scant attention and the curriculum analyses reinforce this. Even the learning outcomes and indicative content for community health care nursing provided by the United Kingdom Central Council largely overlook chronic illness and disability, particularly with respect to the role of the health visitor. It is ironic therefore that this review has suggested that health visitors may have the most significant role in the community environment. The deficits in current provision are such that it is not valid to argue that the health care needs of chronically ill and disabled people are subsumed under those of the general population; their needs must be made explicit and figure far more prominently and cohesively within programmes of preparation for nurses at all levels.

9.3.3   Development of a specialty

The fourth area to which Symington turns attention can be considered as comprising two elements: the shift towards community care and the emergence in many countries of rehabilitation as a distinct specialty. Both are likely to exert increasing influence on the nurse's role in rehabilitation. Community care is now well-established in the UK and consequently far greater emphasis has been placed on a primary care-led NHS. This has been reaffirmed unequivocally in two recent White Papers (Secretary of State for Health, 1996b; 1996c), and presents enormous opportunities for community health care nurses to take a lead role in developing more responsive and holistic services for chronically ill and disabled people and their family carers. To achieve this potential however will mean reconceptualising the roles of such practitioners and reflecting such changes in their educational preparation.

Rehabilitation in the UK, to the extent that it has been perceived as a specialist area of practice at all, has to date largely been the preserve of the therapy disciplines, but this is changing. As already noted there are now standards of practice for rehabilitation nurses (RCN, 1994) and this review has argued that there is both a generic and specific rehabilitative role for nurses. Concurrently however rehabilitation medicine also lays claim to specialty status (Vaughan and Bhakta, 1995) – a development which nursing should heed. There is clearly a need to work as closely as possible with medical and other colleagues, but history would caution that when medicine plays a significant role in any development, this is likely to be the dominant one. The evolution of geriatric medicine and geriatric nursing is a telling example and the parallels between this and the current position in respect of rehabilitation are striking.

Geriatric medicine emerged largely as a response to the therapeutic nihilism regarding the care of older people in the late 1940s and early 1950s. Pioneers such as Marjorie Warren argued that far from being irremediable, many older people could be treated successfully and discharged to home. The introduction of more holistic treatment revolutionised the care older people received and many were indeed successfully discharged from long-stay hospitals. Similarly, nursing research in the UK was spearheaded by practitioners working with older people, particularly Doreen Norton. She contended that care of older people was an area in which nursing could and should excel. Unfortunately this did not materialise, largely because nursing failed to specify what its contribution might be. This was summarised by Wells (1980): *'The central problem in geriatric nursing is the central problem in all of nursing; nurses do not know why they do what they do'.*

Geriatric nursing did not develop a role distinct from, but complementary to, medicine and particularly in long-term care, nurses were left with the tasks that no-one else wanted but without the legitimate authority to act independently, so that patients were subjected to *'aimless residual care'* (Evers, 1991). The analogies between this situation and the general maintenance and carry-on roles ascribed to nurses in rehabilitation are apparent. Furthermore as geriatric medicine struggled to gain acceptance, its early holistic orientation was replaced with a more pragmatic and readily observable criterion of success. Being unable to cure most diseases of old age, yet still being required to achieve a through-put of patients, geriatric medicine substituted a functional model of health for the more traditional medical model (Wilkin and Hughes, 1986), judging success largely by the extent to which function, especially in the activities of daily living, was restored. Again the parallels with current rehabilitation are transparent and if rehabilitation medicine flourishes the push towards observable and measurable outcomes is likely to accelerate.

As illustrated in this review rehabilitation nursing has aspirations towards a more holistic approach which stresses health and wellness rather than disability and illness. Roles such as facilitator and enabler are espoused, but exactly what is to be facilitated or enabled is often not made clear. This is not sufficient and nursing is unlikely to survive and develop by feeding off little other than its own rhetoric. Nurses must be able to specify *what* they are enabling and present a strong case for the value of such interventions. There is abundant literature on the existential and biographical aspects of rehabilitation to provide a sound foundation for practice, but many of these theories need further refinement and empirical testing. At a more focused and grounded level there are numerous opportunities to apply existing or develop new interventions, for example, in areas such as guilt (Flannery, 1990) or helping traumatised patients deal with *'unbearable'* events (Dewar and Morse, 1995). Emerging models such as the *'carers as experts'* framework (Nolan et al, 1996) are also ripe for further development and application. None of these were apparent in the curricula analysed.

The skills level analysis suggested by Twinning (1996) as relating to psychological interventions in rehabilitation has considerable promise to inform nursing education. Broadly this comprises:

- universal skills (markers of good practice relevant to anyone dealing with patients, for example, communication skills)

- specific skills (which can be utilised by most professionals with the relevant training, many forms of counselling fall into this category)

- specialist skills (for complex problems requiring detailed training and knowledge of psychology).

This framework could be allied with a model such as the PLISSIT approach to sexuality developed by Annon (1976) and advocated by Rieve (1989). This composite might then be used to identify which areas of practice fall within the rehabilitative role for nurses, which within a specialist role and which are best left to other disciplines. It is important to consider how such frameworks can be used to help specify the type and level of skills and knowledge needed in various programmes of preparation, how these may be taught and assessed and who should be delivering the content. Only when nursing begins to address issues such as these will it be able to stake a defensible claim to a greater role in the rehabilitative process.

9.3.4 Financial considerations and outcome measures

The fifth of Symington's megatrends highlights concerns over the costs of health care with a resultant focus on efficiency and effectiveness. This factor is also likely to exert a growing influence. One current manifestation of this in the UK is the re-emergence of the pejorative term 'bed-blockers' into mainstream professional discourse. However, a more generalised consequence of the emphasis on costs is the increased interest in outcome measurement; although there are attempts to increase the sensitivity of outcome measures by focusing on handicap rather than simply disability, the overall trend is nevertheless towards functional measures as the primary indicators of successful rehabilitation. The limitations of such a measurement model are compounded by the fact that many instruments lack a sound theoretical basis and are derived primarily from a professional rather than a patient perspective.

Unfortunately the reaction of many nurses is to eschew such instruments altogether, use them in an uncritical and unthinking manner, or develop their own equally superficial measures; none of these reactions is satisfactory. As with most tools there is nothing inherently wrong with measurement if used in the correct context. Indeed it is essential that nurses consider how they can both sensitively measure their own practice and engage in meaningful dialogue with colleagues, particularly medics, about the appropriateness of currently prevalent functional indicators. This requires as a minimum a basic understanding of the principles of scale construction together with, in the case of rehabilitation, an appreciation of some of the relevant theoretical paradigms. Given the prevalence of concepts such as powerlessness, hopelessness and so on in the rehabilitation literature the stress/coping paradigm seems particularly important.

Much is currently written about research appreciation and evidence-based practice, and much of the 'evidence' for rehabilitation (and indeed many other aspects of care) is likely to come via outcome measures. These should therefore form part of the repertoire of all nurses. A basic appreciation is required at pre-registration level which can be built on thereafter. More senior practitioners and nurse researchers have an important role to play in developing measures which result in an individual profile rather than a summary score. Such indices not only provide an initial assessment but also a basis for intervention and subsequent evaluation.

Although the blanket application of a problem-solving approach to care is inappropriate, in situations where problems can be solved it is the model of choice. Nurses need to adopt a more systematic and theoretically valid basis for their problem-solving endeavours and the use of relevant patient and carer centred measures is one such way. The preparation of nurses at both pre- and post-registration levels should facilitate the acquisition of the relevant knowledge and skills. This will also allow the profession to contribute meaningfully to another of Symington's megatrends, the shift from empiricism to applied science and the growth of rehabilitation as a scientific discipline.

9.3.5 New technology

The last area to which Symington calls attention is the growth in assistive technology, and there can be no doubt that this will be an increasingly important component of health care in general and rehabilitation in particular. Whilst Lees and Lepages' (1994) vision of robots replacing care worker may be some way off, the explosion in technology will exert its influence in a myriad of ways from the use of expert systems in education and clinical decision-making (Gonthier and Habel, 1994) to improvements in the quality of life of very frail, house-bound older people (Lawton et al, 1995). As with outcome measures, all nurses need to be aware of the possibilities of assistive technology, while some will make an active contribution to its development. Educational preparation should reflect this.

The use of Symington's (1994) framework has been useful for summarising many of the points raised in the review and highlighting their implications for nurse education. However, the discussion above is not intended to be exhaustive and readers will no doubt identify other areas that reflect their particular interests or concerns. Some other issues not raised so far merit attention. These are now briefly addressed.

9.4 Organisation of care

The first and most obvious of these relates to team-working and the nurse's contribution to the organisation of care. There were encouraging signs from the curriculum analysis that this is now receiving more systematic attention in many programmes at both pre- and post-registration levels. What is required is a thorough understanding, not only of the nurse's role but also of the explicit and implicit assumptions underpinning the practice of other professional disciplines. This should be extended to include professionals working in other agencies, and should consider the barriers to achieving effective teamwork. Nurses also need to be equipped with the communication and assertiveness skills to enable them to take a leadership role in the multidisciplinary team when appropriate. Although the theoretical underpinnings of team-working can be provided in the classroom, suitable practice placements also need to be identified. Moreover in order to get a better grasp of other disciplines, more systematic shared and joint training is needed at all levels. This is particularly important given the increasing complexity of service delivery and the acknowledged need for a more co-ordinated approach (Beardshaw, 1988; Thorne, 1993). As suggested in Figure 6.1 we believe that nurses occupy a unique position, not only by nature of their 24-hour, seven-day input, but also because they have a potential contribution at all stages of rehabilitation, across all environments of care.

Accepting a 24-hour presence as a 'unique' nursing contribution axiomatically mandates a continuation or carry-on role so that the input of other disciplines is maintained in a consistent fashion. This in itself requires both a range of knowledge and skills and better interprofessional communication, and here the nurse's co-ordinating role emerges. However, we believe that there is a superordinate role which is currently lacking and we term this *orchestration*, as we feel this better captures the nuances of rehabilitation in a multiprofessional, multiagency context.

Indeed we would suggest that 'orchestration' provides a useful metaphor to distil the 'essence' of the nurse's *potential* role in rehabilitation. Janesick (1994) used the metaphor of a *'dance'* as a powerful means of conveying the multilayered nature of qualitative research, portraying both dance and qualitative research as expressive, dynamic and interpretative undertakings. We would contend that just as an orchestra achieves harmony despite comprising multiple instruments, each with a defined, but varying, contribution depending on the music being played, successful rehabilitation requires a similar balance. There is clearly a need for rehabilitation to be better orchestrated and nursing, with its input throughout all stages and in all environments, can play a significant part in achieving better, more sensitive and comprehensive rehabilitation that is genuinely in tune with the voices of users and carers. However, this will require a fundamental reorientation of current practice and education.

9.5   Nurse education

A concern raised in this review was Water's (1991; 1996) conclusion that even in areas where nurses are accorded expert status by colleagues, for example, promotion of continence and skin care, they often lack the knowledge to give well-informed care. It seems reasonable to expect that all nurses should have the necessary knowledge and skills in these important areas upon qualification. As a general observation, both the authors who analysed the curricula were struck in certain documents by the plethora of often esoteric and abstract theory (Nolan et al, 1997). In some instances this appeared as a statement of philosophy at the start of a document or module which did not subsequently inform the more detailed content. In other cases the sheer volume of theory included raised questions in the reviewers' minds as to how this could be covered in the allotted hours and, even if it could, what relevance it held for nursing. A sound theoretical basis for practice is essential, but only so much can meaningfully be addressed within a given programme if the requisite ability to apply theory to practice is also to be developed.

In terms of the nurse's role in rehabilitation, the review identified an extensive and growing knowledge base that is of potential relevance. Indeed some of this is essential if even a basic appreciation of the needs of disabled and chronically ill people is to be achieved. Most of this literature was absent from many of the curricula. In already theory-laden programmes it seems paradoxical to suggest the inclusion of yet more, but this is necessary if nurses are to address some of the most pressing, yet neglected, current and future health needs. There is a need to consider the overall balance of the theoretical content of curricula and whether this can be justified and meaningfully addressed within the parameters of a given programme. Explicit links between relevant theories and practice also need to be drawn and greater attention given to how skills are developed. The impetus behind recent reforms of nurse education was to transform nurses from 'doers' into 'knowledgeable doers'. It is questionable if either has been achieved in the areas of chronic illness and disability. Nor is this likely unless greater attention is paid to a number of areas.

As stressed at the start of this report the purpose of the review, in addition to identifying the nurse's current role in rehabilitation, was to begin to construct a framework, based on a wide-ranging consideration of the literature, as to what such a role might be; this was presented in Figure 6.1. There are conceptual lacunae in the framework and both its broad parameters and more detailed content require further refinement and testing. For example, does convalescence represent the nurse's true contribution to rehabilitation (Castledine, 1994) and if so, what part does this once prevalent, but now virtually extinct, component of health care have to play? Considerably more empirical work is needed to expand and test the framework outlined in this report as well as the utility of the *restricted isolated model* and *comprehensive integrative model* as heuristic devices. These have a number of implications for nurse education, some of which have been alluded to above. There is, however, a need for further work in this area and the Board is in the process of commissioning an empirical study to explore the nurse's role in rehabilitation.

Oliver's (1993) apparently simple but ultimately telling question quoted earlier raises fundamental issues about the nature of rehabilitation practice. He goes on to suggest that *'all is not well in the kingdom of rehabilitation'*; after completing this review the authors are inclined to agree. Remedial action is clearly needed. An expansion of the nurse's role in rehabilitation along the lines suggested here could be a step in the right direction, but if initiatives are not to falter then, as Sheppard (1994a; 1994b) suggests, the nursing contribution to rehabilitation must be made more visible, it is no longer sufficient to maintain that much of what nursing does constitutes *'invisible mending'* (RCN, 1996). We suggest rather that visibility needs to occur at a number of levels.

First, the nurse's current role in rehabilitation needs to be recognised and more clearly articulated both within and outwith the profession. For this to be achieved the role has to figure more prominently in programmes of preparation. Second, the dimensions of an expanded role in rehabilitation need to be explored. To achieve this nurses must create real (as opposed to rhetorical) partnerships with disabled and chronically ill people. Practitioners need to be alerted to the possibilities for such partnerships and their imaginations fired to pursue them. This will not occur until issues surrounding rehabilitation, disability and chronic illness have a more prominent place in curricula – currently they are all but invisible. Last, but by no means least, it has to be realised that vague notions of empowerment, enablement and holistic care cannot sustain a profession. If nursing is serious in its intent to address the health care needs of the population then, for a significant and growing section of that population, this will mean grappling with the more diffuse existential, biographical and temporal dimensions of rehabilitation and articulating clearly, both to fellow professionals and disabled people and their carers, what it is that nursing has to offer.

REFERENCES

Ahern, M.J., McFarlane, A.C., Leslie, A. et al (1995) Illness behaviour in patients with arthritis. *Annals of Rheumatic Disease,* 54, 245-50.

Akridge, R.L. (1986) A community model of habilitation/rehabilitation. *Journal of Rehabilitative Administration*, 10, 3, 81-85.

Allen, I., Levin, E., Siddell, M., Vetter, N. (1983) The elderly and their informal carers. In: Allen, I., Levin, E., Siddell, M., Vetter, N. (Eds) *Elderly People in the Community: Their service needs.* London: HMSO.

Anderson, R. (1988) The quality of life of stroke patients and their carers. In: Robinson, I. and Bury, M. (Eds) *Living with Chronic Illness*. London: Unwin Hyman.

Anderson, J.M. (1991) Immigrant women speak of chronic illness: the social context of devalued self. *Journal of Advanced Nursing*, 16, 710-717.

Anderton, J.M., Elfert, H., Lai, M. (1989) Ideology in the clinical context: chronic illness, ethnicity and the discourse of normalisation. *Sociology of Health and Illness*, 11, 3, 253-278.

Andrews, K. (1987) *Rehabilitation of Older Adults*. London: Edward Arnold.

Annon, J. (1976) The PLISSIT Model: a proposed conceptual scheme for the behavioural treatment of sexual problems. *Journal of Sex Education and Therapy*, 2, 1.

Antonovsky, A. (1987) *Unravelling the Mystery of Health*. San Francisco: Jossey-Bass.

Archbold, P.G., Stewart, B.J., Greenlick, M.R., Harvath, T.A. (1992) The clinical assessment of mutuality and preparedness in family caregivers of frail older people. In: Funk, S.G., Tornquist, E.M.T., Champagne, S.T., Wiese, R.A. (Eds) *Key Aspects of Elder Care: Managing falls, incontinence and cognitive impairment*. New York: Springer.

Asvall, J.E. (1992) Foreword. In: Kaplun, A. (Ed.) *Health Promotion and Chronic Illness: Discovering a new quality of health*. Copenhagen: WHO Regional Publications. European Series No. 44.

Bach, M. and Rioux, M.H. (1996) Social well-being: a framework for quality of life research. In: Renwick, R., Brown, I., Nagler, M. (Eds) *Quality of Life in Health Promotion and Rehabilitation: Conceptual approaches, issues and applications*. Thousand Oaks, California: Sage.

Badley, E.M. and Lee, J. (1987) Impairment, disability and the ICIDH (International Classification of Impairments, Disabilities and Handicaps) Model I: the relationship between impairment and disability. *International Rehabilitation Medicine*, 8, 113-117.

Badley, E.M., Lee, J., Wood, P.H.N. (1987) Impairment, disability and the ICIDH Model II: the nature of the underlying conditions and patterns of impairment. *International Rehabilitation Medicine*, 8, 118-124.

Badley, E.M. (1995) The genesis of handicap: definitions, models of disablement and role of external factors. *Disability and Rehabilitation*, 17, 2, 53-62.

Baggerley, J., Belmosto, L., Drinkwater, J., Master, M. (1995) Patients' readiness for scheduled therapies: nursing's positive contribution. *Rehabilitation Nursing*, 20, 3, 161-163.

Bailey, R. and Clarke, M. (1989) *Stress and Coping in Nursing*. London: Chapman Hall.

Baines, E.M. and Oglesby, F.M. (1991) Conceptualisation of chronicity in aging. In: Baines, E.M. (Ed.) *Perspectives on Gerontological Nursing*. Newbury Park: Sage.

Baker, C. and Stern, P.N. (1993) Finding meaning in chronic illness as the key to self-care. *Canadian Journal of Nursing Research*, 25, 2, 23-36.

Baker, M., Fardell, J., Jones, B. (1997) *Disability and Rehabilitation: Survey of education needs of health and social service professionals – the case for action*. London: Disability and Rehabilitation, Open Learning Project.

Barber, G. (1995) Searching the therapy and rehabilitation literature. *British Journal of Therapy and Rehabilitation*, 2, 4, 203-208.

Barnard, D. (1995) Chronic illness and the dynamics of hoping. In: Toombs, S.K., Barnard, D., Carson, R. (Eds) *Chronic Illness: From experience to policy*. Bloomington: Indiana University Press.

References

Barnes, M.P. (1993) Organisation of rehabilitation services. In: Greenwood, R., Barnes, M.P., McMillan, T.M., Ward, C.D. (Eds) *Neurological Rehabilitation*. Edinburgh: Churchill Livingstone.

Barnitt, R. and Pomeroy, V. (1995) A holistic approach to rehabilitation. *British Journal of Therapy and Rehabilitation*, **2**, 2, 87-92.

Beardshaw, V. (1988) *Last in the List: Community services for people with physical disabilities*. London: King's Fund Institute.

Beck, R.J. (1994) Encouragement as a vehicle to empowerment in counselling: an existential perspective. *Journal of Rehabilitation*, **60**, 3, 6-11.

Becker, G. and Kaufman, S. (1988) Old age, rehabilitation and research: a review of the issues. *Gerontologist*, **28**, 4, 459-468.

Beckmann, J. and Ditlev, G. (1992) Conceptual views on quality of life. In: Kaplun, A. (Ed.) *Health Promotion and Chronic Illness: Discovering a new quality of health*. Copenhagen: WHO Regional Publications, European Series, No. 44.

Bell, R. and Gibbons, S. (1989) *Working with Carers: Information and training for work with informal carers of elderly people*. London: Health Education Authority.

Benner, P. (1984) *From Novice to Expert: Excellence and power in clinical nursing practice*. Menlo Park, California: Addison-Wesley.

Benner, P. and Wruebel, J. (1989) *The Primacy of Caring: Stress and coping in health and illness*. Menlo Park, California: Addison-Wesley.

Ben-Sira, Z. (1989) Potency: a readjustment promoting link in the rehabilitation of the disabled person. *Sociology of Health and Illness*, **11**, 1, 41-61.

Benson, L. and Ducanies, A. (1995) Nurses' perceptions of their role and role conflicts. *Rehabilitation Nursing*, **20**, 4, 204-211.

Biegel, D.E., Soles, E., Schulz, R. (1991) *Family Caregiving in Chronic Illness*. Newbury Park: Sage.

Blaxter, M. (1976) *The Meaning of Disability*. London: Heinemann Educational Books.

Bloch, D.A. (1993) Foreword. In: Rolland, J.S. (1994) *Families, Illness and Disability: An integrative treatment model*. New York: Basic Books.

Bodenhamer, E., Achterberg Lawlis, J., Kevorkian, G. et al (1983) Staff and patient perceptions of the psychosocial concerns of spinal cord injured persons. *American Journal of Physical Medicine*, **62**, 182-193.

Booth, A. (1996) In search of the evidence: informing effective practice. *Journal of Clinical Effectiveness*, **1**, 1, 25-29.

Bowles, L., Oliver, N., Stanley, S. (1995) A fresh approach. *Nursing Times*, **91**, 1, 40-41.

Bowling, A. (1991) *Measuring Health: A review of quality of life measurement scales*. Milton Keynes: Open University Press.

Bowling, A. (1995) *Measuring Disease: A review of disease-specific quality of life measurement scales*. Buckingham: Open University Press.

Boynton De Sepulveda, L.I. and Chang, B. (1994) Effective coping with stroke disability in a community setting: the development of a causal model. *Journal of Neuroscience Nursing*, **26**, 4, 193-203.

Braden, C.J. (1990) Learned self-help response to chronic illness experience: a test of three alternative learning theories. *Scholarly Inquiry for Nursing Practice*, **4**, 1, 23-41.

Braden, C.J. (1993) Research program on learned response to chronic illness experience: self help model. *Holistic Nurse Practice*, **8**, 1, 38-44.

Braithwaite, V.A. (1990) *Bound to Care*. Sydney: Allen and Unwin.

Brandsma, J.W., Kakerveld-Heyl, K., van Ravensberg, C.D., Heakens, Y.F. (1995) Reflection on the definition of impairment and disability as defined by the WHO. *Disability and Rehabilitation*, **17**, 314, 119-127.

Brandstädter, J. (1995) *Maintaining a Sense of Control and Self-esteem in Later Life: Protective mechanisms*. Paper presented at III European Congress of Gerontology, Amsterdam, 30 August - 2 September 1995.

Brandstädter, J., Wentura, D., Greve, W. (1993) Adoptive resources of the aging self: outlines of an emergent perspective. *International Journal of Behavioural Development*, **16**, 2, 323-349.

Brandstädter, J. and Greve, W. (1994) The aging self: stabilising and protective processes. *Developmental Review*, **14**, 52-80.

Brazier, H. and Begley, C.M. (1996) Selecting a database for literature searches in nursing: MEDLINE or CINAHL? *Journal of Advanced Nursing*, **24**, 868-875.

Brillhart, B. and Stewart, A. (1989) Education as the key to rehabilitation. *Nursing Clinics of North America*, **24**, 3, 675-680.

Brody, E.M. (1995) Prospects for family caregiving: response to change, continuity and diversity. In: Kane, R.A. and Penrod, J.D. (Eds) *Family Caregiving in an Ageing Society*. Thousand Oaks, California: Sage.

Brown, J. (1993) Coping with stress: the beneficial role of positive illusions. In: Turnbull, A.P., Patterson, J.M., Behr, S.K. et al (Eds) *Cognitive Coping, Families and Disability*. Baltimore: Paul H Brookes.

Brown, S. and Williams, A. (1995) Women's experiences of rheumatoid arthritis. *Journal of Advanced Nursing*, **21**, 695-701.

Brown, I., Renwick, R., Nagler, M. (1996) The centrality of quality of life in health promotion and rehabilitation. In: Renwick, R., Brown, I., Nagler, M. (Eds) *Quality of Life in Health Promotion and Rehabilitation: Conceptual approaches, issues and applications*. Thousand Oaks, California: Sage.

Brummel-Smith, K. (1993) Research in rehabilitation. *Clinics in Geriatric Medicine*, **9**, 4, 895-904.

Bryant, E.T. (1995) Acute rehabilitation – an outcome orientated model. In: Landrum, P.K., Schmidt, N.D., McLean, A. Jr (Eds) *Outcome Orientated Rehabilitation: Principles, strategies and tools for effective programme management*. Gaithenburg: Aspen Publications.

Burggraf, V. and Barry, R. (1995) Long term care: providing for those with disability and chronic illness. *Journal of Gerontological Nursing*, October 1995, **21**, 10, 31-35.

Burnham, J. and Shearer, B. (1993) Comparison of CINAHL, EMBASE and MEDLINE databases for the nurse researcher. *Medical Reference Services Quarterly*, **12**, 3, 45-57.

Burr, W.R., Klein, S.R. and Associates (1994) *Re-examining Family Stress: New theory and research*. Thousand Oaks, California: Sage.

Bury, M. (1982) Chronic illness as biographical disruption. *Sociology of Health and Illness*, **4**, 2, 167-182.

Cairns, D. and Baker, J. (1993) Adjustment to spinal cord injury: a review of coping styles contributing to the process. *Journal of Rehabilitation*, **59**, 30-33.

Carpenter, C. (1994) The experience of spinal cord injury: the individual's perspective – implications for rehabilitation practice. *Physical Therapy*, **74**, 7, 614-627.

Carricaburu, D. and Pierret, J. (1995) From biographical disruption to biographical reinforcement: the case of HIV positive men. *Sociology of Health and Illness*, **17**, 1, 65-92.

Carson, R.A. (1995) Beyond respect to recognition and due regard. In: Toombs S.K., Barnard, D., Carson, R.A. (Eds) *Chronic Illness: from experience to policy*. Bloomington: Indiana University Press.

Castledine, G. (1994) The value of convalescent care. *British Journal of Nursing*, **3**, 14, 728-729.

Charmaz, K. (1983) Loss of self – a fundamental form of suffering in the chronically ill. *Sociology of Health and Illness*, **5**, 2, 168-195.

Charmaz, K. (1987) Struggling for self: identify levels of the chronically ill. *Sociology of Health Care*, **6**, 283-321.

Chiou, L. and Burnett, C.N. (1985) Values of activities of daily living: a survey of stroke patients and their home therapists. *Physical Therapy*, **65**, 901-906.

Clark, P.G. (1995) Quality of life, values and teamwork in geriatric care: do we communicate what we mean? *Gerontologist*, **35**, 3, 402-411.

Coates, V.E. and Boore, J.R.P. (1995) Self-management of chronic illness and implications for nursing. *International Journal of Nursing Studies*, **32**, 6, 628-640.

Cohen, M.H. (1993) The unknown and the unachievable – managing sustained uncertainty. *Western Journal of Nursing Research*, **15**, 1, 77-96.

Conwill, J. (1993) Understanding and combating helplessness. *Rehabilitation Nursing*, **18**, 6, 388-394, 399.

References

Cope, D.N. and Sundance, P. (1995) Conceptualising clinical outcomes. In: Landrum, P.K., Schmidt, N.D., McLean, A. Jr (Eds) *Outcome Orientated Rehabilitation: Principles, strategies and tools for effective program management*. Gaithenburg: Aspen Publications.

Corbin, J.M. and Strauss, A. (1988) *Unending work and care: Managing chronic illness at home*. San Francisco: Jossey-Bass.

Corbin, J.M. and Strauss, A. (1991) A nursing model for chronic illness management based upon the trajectory framework. *Scholarly Inquiry for Nursing Practice*, **5**, 3, 155-174.

Corbin, J.M. and Strauss, A. (1992) A nursing model for chronic illness management based upon the trajectory framework. In: Woog, E. (Ed.) *The Chronic Illness Trajectory Framework*. New York: Springer.

Cowley, S. (1995) Health as a process: a health visiting perspective. *Journal of Advanced Nursing*, **22**, 433-441.

Curry, R.L. (1995) The exceptional family: walking the edge of tragedy and transformation. In: Toombs, S.K., Barnard, D., Carson, R.A. (1995) *Chronic Illness: From experience to policy*. Bloomington: Indiana University Press.

Dangoor, N. and Florian, V. (1994) Women with chronic physical disabilities: correlates of their long-term psychological adaptation. *International Journal of Rehabilitation Research*, **17**, 159-168.

Davies, M.C. (1994) The rehabilitation nurses role in spiritual care. *Rehabilitation Nursing*, **19**, 5, 298-301.

Davies, S.M. (1995) An investigation into nurses' understanding of health education and health promotion within a neuro-rehabilitation setting. *Journal of Advanced Nursing*, **21**, 951-959.

Day, H. and Jankey, S.G. (1996) Lessons from the literature: towards a holistic model of quality of life. In: Renwick, R., Brown, I., Nagler, M. (Eds) *Quality of Life in Health Promotion and Rehabilitation: Conceptual approaches, issues and applications*. Thousand Oakes, California: Sage.

Dean-Baar, S.L. (1994) Development of the Arthritis Health Belief Inventory. *Rehabilitation Nursing Research*, **3**, 111-21,129.

Dejong, G. and Sutton, J.P. (1995) Rehabilitation 2000: The evolution of medical rehabilitation in American health care. In: Landrum, P.K., Schmidt, N.D., McLean, A. Jr (Eds) *Outcome Orientated Rehabilitation: Principles, strategies and tools for effective program management*. Gaithenburg: Aspen Publications.

Dewar, A.L. and Morse, J.M. (1995) Unbearable incidents – failure to endure the experience of illness. *Journal of Advanced Nursing*, **22**, 5, 957-964.

Dewis, M.E. (1989) Spinal cord injured adolescents and young adults: the meaning of body changes. *Journal of Advanced Nursing*, **14**, 389-396.

Dickson, H.G. (1996) Problems with ICIDH definition of impairment. *Disability and Rehabilitation*, **18**, 1, 52-54.

Dijkers, M. and Cushman, L.A. (1990) Differences between rehabilitation disciplines in views of depression in spinal cord injury patients. *Paraplegia*, **28**, 380-391.

Diller, L. (1990) Fostering the interdisciplinary team, fostering research in a society in transition. *Archives of Physical Medicine and Rehabilitation*, **71**, 275-278.

Doherty, W.J. and Campbell, T.L. (1988) *Families and Health*. Newbury Park: Sage.

Donnelly, G.F. (1995) Chronicity, concept and reality. *Holistic Nursing Practice*, **8**, 1, 1-7.

Doolittle, N.D. (1988) Stroke recovery: review of the literature and suggestions for future research. *Journal of Neuroscience Nursing*, **20**, 169-173.

Doolittle, N.D. (1991) Clinical ethnography of lacunar stroke: implications for acute care. *Journal of Neuroscience Nursing*, **23**, 235-240.

Doolittle, N.D. (1992) The experience of recovery following lacunar stroke. *Rehabilitation Nursing*, **17**, 122-126.

Doolittle, N.D. (1994) A clinical ethnography of stroke recovery. In: Benner, P. (Ed.) *Interpretive Phenomenology Embodiment, Caring and Ethics in Health and Illness*. Newbury Park: Sage.

Downe-Wamboldt, B.L. and Melanson, P.M. (1995) Emotions, coping, and psychological well-being in elderly people with arthritis. *Western Journal of Nursing Research*, **17**, 250-265.

Dutton, R. (1995) *Clinical Reasoning in Physical Disabilities*. Baltimore: Williams and Wilkins.

Dyck, I. (1995) Hidden geographies: the changing lifeworlds of women with multiple sclerosis. *Social Science and Medicine*, **40**, 307-320.

Eraut, M. (1994) *Developing Professional Knowledge and Competence*. London: The Falmer Press.

Eubanks, P. (1990) Chronic care: a future delivery model. *Hospitals*, **64**, 6, 42-46.

Evans, R.L., Connis, R.T., Hendrick, R.D., Haselkem, J.K. (1995) Multidisciplinary rehabilitation vs medical care: a meta-analysis. *Social Science and Medicine*, **40**, 12, 1699-1706.

Evers, H.K. (1981) Multidisciplinary teams in geriatric wards: myth or reality? *Journal of Advanced Nursing*, **6**, 205-214.

Evers, H.K. (1991) Care of the elderly sick in the UK. In: Redfern, S.J. (Ed.) *Nursing Elderly People*. Edinburgh: Churchill Livingstone.

Fairhurst, E. (1981) What do you do? Multiple realities in occupational therapy and rehabilitation. In: Atkinson, P., Health, C. (Eds) *Medical Work: Realities and routines*. Farnborough: Gower.

Fallowfield, D.L. (1990) *The Quality of Life: The missing measurement in health care*. London: Souvenier Press.

Farran, C.J., Keith, K.A., Popovich, J.M. (1995) *Hope and Hopelessness: Critical clinical constructs*. Thousand Oakes, California: Sage.

Felce, D. and Perry, J. (1996) Exploring current conceptions of quality of life: a model for people with and without disabilities. In: Renwick, R., Brown, I., Nagler, M. (Eds) *Quality of Life in Health Promotion and Rehabilitation: Conceptual approaches, issues and applications*. Thousand Oakes, California: Sage.

Felton, B.J., Revenson, T.A., Hinrichsen, G.A. (1984) Coping with chronic illness: a study of illness controllability and the influence of coping strategies on psychological adjustment among chronically ill adults. *Journal of Consulting and Clinical Psychology*, **52**, 3, 343-353.

Fife, B.L. (1995) The measurement of meaning in illness. *Social Science and Medicine*, **40**, 8, 1021-1028.

Finkelstein, V. (1981) *Disability and Professional Attitudes*. Seven Oaks: Naidex Conventions.

Finkelstein, V. and Stuart, O. (1996) Developing new services. In: Hales, G. (Ed.) *Beyond Disability: Toward an enabling society*. London: Sage (in association with OU).

Fitzgerald, M.H. and Paterson, K.A. (1995) The hidden disability dilemma for the preservation of self. *Journal of Occupational Science*, **2**, 13-21.

Fitzpatrick, R. (1996) Patient-centred approaches to the evaluation of health care. In: Fulford, K.W.M., Ersser, S., Hope, T. (Eds) *Essential Practice in Patient Centred Care*. Oxford: Blackwell Science.

Flannery, J. (1990) Guilt: a crisis within a crisis... a catastrophic neurologic event. *Journal of Neuroscience Nursing*, **22**, 2, 92-99.

Folden, S.L. (1994) Managing the effects of a stroke: the first months. *Rehabilitation Nursing Research*, **3**, 79-85.

Folkman, S. and Lazarus, R.S. (1985) If it changes it must be a process: a study of emotion and coping during three stages of a college examination. *Journal of Personality and Social Psychology*, **48**, 150-70.

Ford, J.S. (1989) Living with a history of a heart attack: a human science investigation. *Journal of Advanced Nursing*, **14**, 173-179.

Forsythe, E. (1988) *MS: Explaining sickness and health*. London: Faber and Faber.

Friedland, J. and McColl, M. (1992) Disability and depression – some etiologic considerations. *Social Science and Medicine*, **34**, 4, 395-403.

Fulford, K.W.M. (1996) Concepts of disease and the meaning of patient centred care. In: Fulford, K.W.M., Ersser, S., Hope, T. (Eds) *Essential Practice in Patient Centred Care*. Oxford: Blackwell Science.

Funk, S.G., Tornquist, E.M., Champagne, M.T., Wiese, R.A. (1993) (Eds) *Key Aspects of Caring for the Chronically Ill: Hospital and home*. New York: Springer.

Gale, G. and Gaylard, J. (1996) The role of the nurse in rehabilitation of older people. In: Squires, A.J. (Ed.) *Rehabilitation of Older People: A handbook for the MDT* (2nd Edn). London: Chapman Hall.

Garrison, S.J. (1995) (Ed.) *Handbook of Physical Medicine and Rehabilitation Basics*. Philadelphia: JB Lippincott Co.

George, J. and Young, J. (1996) Rehabilitation and elderly ethnic minorities. In: Squires, A.J. (Ed.) *Rehabilitation of Older People: A handbook for the MDT* (2nd Edn). London: Chapman Hall.

References

Gerhardt, U. (1989) *Ideas About Illness: An intellectual and political history of medical sociology.* Basingstoke: MacMillan.

Gerhardt, U. (1990) Qualitative research on chronic illness – the issue and the story. *Social Science and Medicine,* **30**, 11, 1149-1159.

Gibbon, B. (1991) A re-assessment of nurses' attitudes towards stroke patients in general medical wards. *Journal of Advanced Nursing,* **16**, 1336-1342.

Gibbon, B. and Thompson, A. (1992) The role of the nurse in rehabilitation. *Nursing Standard,* **6**, 36, 32-35.

Gibbons, K.B., Salter, J.P., Piece, L.L., Govoni, A.L. (1995) A model for professional rehabilitation nursing practice. *Rehabilitation Nursing,* **20**, 1, 23-28, 36.

Gillies, D.A. (1988) Role supplementation to overcome intrafamilial role insufficiency following physical disability. *Rehabilitation Nursing,* **13**, 19-22.

Given, B.A. and Given, C.W. (1991) Family caregivers for the elderly. In: Fitzpatrick, J., Tauton, R., Jacox, A. (Eds) *Annual Review of Nursing Research* (vol. 9). New York: Springer.

Glaser, B. and Strauss, A. (1967) *The Discovery of Grounded Theory.* Chicago: Aldine.

Glass, T.A. and Maddox, G.L. (1992) The quality and quantity of social support: stroke recovery as psycho-social transition. *Social Science and Medicine,* **34**, 1249-1261.

Glueckauf, R.L., Sechrest, L.B., Bord, G.R., McDonel, E.G. (1993) (Eds) *Improving Assessment in Rehabilitation and Health.* Newbury Park: Sage.

Gonthier, R. and Habel, M. (1994) Using algorithms in rehabilitation nursing: an educational strategy. *Rehabilitation Nursing,* **19**, 134-140, 190.

Grainger, C.V. (1986) Outcome of comprehensive medical rehabilitation: an analysis based upon the impairment, disability and handicap model. *International Rehabilitation Medicine,* 7, 45-50.

Grainger, C.V., Kelly-Hayes, M., Johnston, M. et al (1996) Quality and outcome measures for medical rehabilitation. In: Buschbacher, R.M., Dumitru, D., Johnson, E.W. et al (Eds) *Physical Medicine and Rehabilitation.* Philadelphia: Saunders.

Grenville, J. and Lyne, P. (1995) Patient-centred evaluation and rehabilitative care. *Journal of Advanced Nursing,* **22**, 6, 965-972.

Gubrium, J. (1995) Taking stock. *Qualitative Health Research,* **5**, 3, 267-269.

Gullickson, C. (1993) My death nearing its future: a heideggerian hermeneutical analysis of the lived experience with chronic illness. *Journal of Advanced Nursing,* **18**, 1386-1392.

Guthrie, S. and Harvey, A. (1994) Motivation and its influence on outcomes in rehabilitation. *Reviews in Clinical Gerontology,* **4**, 235-243.

Häggström, T., Axelsson, K., Norberg, A. (1994) The experience of living with stroke sequelae illuminated by means of stories and metaphors. *Qualitative Health Research,* **4**, 321-337.

Hainsworth, M.A., Eakes, G.G., Burke, M.L. (1994) Coping with chronic sorrow. *Issues in Mental Health Nursing,* **15**, 59-66.

Halbertsma, J. (1995) The ICIDH: health problems from a medical and social perspective. *Disability and Rehabilitation,* **17**, 314, 128-134.

Halstead, L.S. (1976) Team care in chronic illness: a critical review of the literature of the past 25 years. *Archives of Physical Medicine and Rehabilitation,* **57**, 507-511.

Halstead, L.S., Rintala, D.H., Kanellos, M. et al (1986) The innovative rehabilitation team: an experiment in team building. *Archives of Physical Medicine and Rehabilitation,* **67**, 357-361.

Harvath, T.A., Archbold, P.G., Stewart, B.J. et al (1994) Establishing partnerships with family caregivers: local and cosmopolitan knowledge. *Journal of Gerontological Nursing,* **20**, 2, 29-35.

Harwood, R.H., Jitapunkul, S., Dickinson, E., Ebrahim, S. (1994) Measuring handicap: motives, methods and a model. *Quality in Health Care,* **3**, 53-57.

Hastings, M. (1996) Team working in rehabilitation. In: Squires, A.J. (Ed.) *Rehabilitation of Older People: A handbook for the MDT* (2nd Edn). London: Chapman Hall.

Hawthorne, M.H. (1991) Using the trajectory framework: reconceptualizing cardiac illness. *Scholarly Inquiry for Nursing Practice,* **5**, 185-195.

Helmericks, S.G., Nelsen, R.L., Unnithan, N.P. (1991) The researcher, the topic and the literature: a procedure for systematising literature searches. *Journal of Applied Behavioural Science,* **27**, 3, 285-294.

Henderson, V. (1980) Preserving the essence of nursing in a technological age. *Journal of Advanced Nursing*, 5, 245-260.

Henderson, E.J., Morrison, J.A., Young, E.A., Pentland, B. (1990) The nurse in rehabilitation after severe brain injury. *Clinical Rehabilitation*, 4, 167-172.

Henderson, C.M., Rhodes, R., Ward, A.S. (1995) A rehabilitation practicum for nursing students. *Rehabilitation Nursing*, 20, 2, 109-110.

Henwood, M. (1992) *Through a Glass Darkly: Community care and elderly people*. London: King's Fund Institute, Research Report No. 14.

Hermann, C.P. and Bays, C.L. (1994) Professional rehabilitation nursing: an elective course for nursing students. *Rehabilitation Nursing*, 19, 160-162, 168.

Hershenson, D.B. (1990) A theoretical model for rehabilitation counselling. *Rehabilitation Counselling Bulletin*, 33, 4, 268-278.

Hickman, M., Drummond, N., Grimshaw, J. (1994) A taxonomy of shared care for chronic disease. *Journal of Public Health Medicine*, 16, 4, 447-454.

Higgins, P.C. (1985) *The Rehabilitation Detectives: Doing human services work*. London: Sage.

Hobus, R. (1992) Literature: a dimension of nursing therapists. In: Miller; J.F. (Ed.) *Coping with Chronic Illness: Overseeing powerlessness* (2nd Edn). Philadelphia: FA Davies.

Hoeman, S.P. (1996) Conceptual bases for rehabilitation nursing. In: Hoeman, S.P. (Ed.) *Rehabilitation Nursing: Process and application* (2nd Edn). St Louis: Mosby.

Hollingbery, R (1994) Elderly people's integrated care system (EPICS) and shared care knowledge. *BASELINE*, June 1994, No. 55, 23-41.

Hosking, S. (1984) Rheumatoid arthritis – fundamental nursing care. *Nursing*, 2, 900-901.

Howell, S.L. (1994) A theoretical model for caring for women with chronic non-malignant pain. *Qualitative Health Research*, 4, 1, 94-122.

Hunter, D.J. and Wistow, G. (1991) *EPICS: An organisational, policy and practice review*. Leeds: Nuffield Institute for Health Services Studies, University of Leeds.

Hunt-Raleigh, E.D. (1992) Sources of hope in chronic illness. *Oncology Nursing Forum*, 19, 3, 443-448.

Hymovich, D.P. and Hagopian, G.A. (1992) *Chronic illness in children and adults: A psychosocial approach*. Philadelphia: WB Saunders.

Ingebretsen, R. and Solen, P.E. (1995) *Attachment, Loss and Coping in Caring for a Dementing Spouse*. Paper presented at III European Congress of Gerontology, Amsterdam, 30 August - 2 September 1995.

Ireys, H.T., Werthamer-Larsson, L.A., Kolonder, K.B., Gross, S.S. (1994) Mental health of young adults with chronic illness: the mediating effect of perceived impact. *Journal of Paediatric Psychology*, 19, 2, 205-222.

Irwin, P. (1996) The role of the nurse in stroke. In: Wolfe, C., Rudd, T., Beech, R. (Eds) *Stroke Services and Research*. London: Stroke Association.

Jackson, M.F. (1984) Geriatric rehabilitation on an acute care medical unit. *Journal of Advanced Nursing*, 5, 441-448.

Jackson, O.S. (1987) Basic principles in rehabilitation. *Clinical Physical Therapy*, 14, 1-22.

James, J.E. and Minichiello, V. (1994) Disability and rehabilitation in older persons: biopsychosocial foundations. *Disability and Rehabilitation*, 16, 3, 95-97.

Janesick, V.J. (1994) The dance of qualitative research design: metaphor, methodology and meaning. In: Denzin, N.K. and Lincoln, Y.S. (Eds) *Handbook of Qualitative Research*. Thousand Oakes, California: Sage.

Jelles, F., Van Bennekom, C.A.M., Lankhorst, G.J. (1995) The interdisciplinary team conference in rehabilitation medicine. In: Van Bennekom, C.A.M. and Jelles, F. (Eds) *Rehabilitation Activities Profile*. Amsterdam: Vrije Universiteit.

Jensen, L.A. and Allen, M.N. (1994) A synthesis of qualitative research on wellness – illness. *Qualitative Health Research*, 4, 4, 349-369.

Johnson, J.L. (1991) Learning to live again: the process of adjustment following a heart attack. In: Morse, J.M., Johnson, L.J. (Eds) *The Illness Experience Dimensions of Suffering*. Newbury Park: Sage.

References

Johnson, J.L. and Morse, J.M. (1990) Regaining control: the process of adjustment after myocardial infarction. *Heart and Lung: Journal of Critical Care*, **19**, 126-135.

Johnson, J. (1995) Achieving effective rehabilitation outcomes: does the nurse have a role? *British Journal of Therapy and Rehabilitation*, **2**, 3, 113-118.

Joseph, C.L. and Wanlass, W. (1993) Rehabilitation in the nursing home. *Clinics in Geriatric Medicine*, **9**, 4, 859-871.

Kaplun, A. (1964) *The Conduct of Inquiry: Methodology for behavioural sciences*. San Francisco: Chandler Publishing.

Keane, S.M., Chastain, B., Rudisill, K. (1987) Caring: nurse-patient perceptions. *Rehabilitation Nursing*, **12**, 4, 182-184.

Keir, D. (1996) Rehabilitation: complex values of a limitless team. In: Squires, A.J. (Ed.) *Rehabilitation of Older People: A handbook for the MDT* (2nd Edn). London: Chapman Hall.

Keith, R.A. (1991) The comprehensive treatment teams in rehabilitation. *Archives of Physical Medicine and Rehabilitation*, **72**, 269-274.

Keith, R.A. (1995) Conceptual basis of outcome measures. *American Journal of Physical Medicine and Rehabilitation*, 77, 73-80.

Keith, R.A. and Lipsey, M.W. (1993) The role of theory in rehabilitation assessment treatment and outcomes. In: Glueckauf, R.L., Sechrest, L.B., Bond, G.R., McDonel, E.G. (Eds) *Improving Assessment in Rehabilitation and Health*. Newbury Park: Sage.

Kelly-Hayes, M. (1996) Functional evaluation. In: Hoeman, S.P. (Ed.) *Rehabilitation Nursing: Process and application* (2nd Edn). St Louis: Mosby.

Kemp, B.J. (1988) Motivation rehabilitation and ageing: a conceptual model. *Geriatric Rehabilitation*, **3**, 3, 41-51.

Kemp, B.J. (1993) Psychological care of older rehabilitation patient. *Clinics in Geriatric Medicine*, **9**, 4, 841-857.

Kleinmann, A. (1995) The social course of chronic illness: delegitimation, resistance and transformation in North American and Chinese societies. In: Toombs, S.K., Darnard, D., Carson, R.A. (Eds) *Chronic Illness: From experience to policy*. Bloomington: Indiana University Press.

Knafl, K.A. and Deatrick, J.A. (1990) Family management style: concept analysis and development. *Journal of Paediatric Nursing*, **5**, 1, 4-14.

Knight, B.G. (1996) *Psychotherapy with Older Adults* (2nd Edn). Thousand Oaks: Sage.

Kraft, G.H., Freal, J.E., Coryell J K (1986) Disability, disease duration, and rehabilitation service needs in multiple sclerosis – patient perspectives. *Archives of Physical Medicine and Rehabilitation*, **67**, 164-168.

Krippendorf, K. (1980) *Content Analysis: An introduction to its methodology*. Beverly Hills: Sage.

Lafaille, R. (1992) Training: needs and possibilities. In: Kaplun, A. (Ed.) *Health Promotion and Chronic Illness: Discovering a new quality of health*. Copenhagen: WHO Regional Publications. European Series No. 44.

Lafferty, G. (1996) Community-based alternatives to hospital rehabilitation services: a review of the evidence and suggestions for approaching future evolution. *Reviews in Clinical Gerontology*, **6**, 2, 183-194.

Laman, H. and Lankhorst, G.J. (1994) Subjective weighting of disability: an approach to quality of life assessment in rehabilitation. *Disability and Rehabilitation*, **16**, 4, 198-204.

Lamb, G.S. and Stempel, J.E. (1994) Nurse case management from the client's view: growing as insider-expert. *Nursing Outlook*, **42**, 7-13.

Lambert, V.A. (1991) Arthritis. *Annual Review of Nursing Research* (vol. 9). New York: Springer.

Landrum, P.K., Schmidt, N.D., McLean, A. Jr (1995) *Outcome-orientated Rehabilitation: Principles, strategies and tools for effective program management*. Gaithenburg: Aspen Publications.

Langhorne, P., Williams, B.O., Gilchrist, W., Howie, K. (1993) Do stroke units save lives? *Lancet*, **342**, 8868, 395-398.

Lankhorst, S.J., Jelles, F., Van Bennekom, C.A.M. (1995) *Rehabilitation Activity Profile: Manual and description*. Amsterdam: Vrije Universiteit.

Larsson, S. (1995) Vocational rehabilitation: a Swedish model for assessment, treatment, training and reinstatement. *Work*, **5**, 3, 205-121.

Lawton, M.P., Moss, M., Dunamel, L.M. (1995) The quality of life among elderly care receivers. *Journal of Applied Gerontology*, **14**, 2, 150-71.

Lazarus, R.S. (1992) Coping with the stress of illness. In: Kaplun, A. (Ed.) *Health Promotion and Chronic Illness: Discovering a new quality of health*. Copenhagen: WHO Regional Publications, European Series No. 44.

Lazarus, R.S. (1993) Coping theory and research: past, recent and future. *Psychosomatic Medicine*, **55**, 234-47.

Lazarus, R.S. and Folkman, S. (1984) *Stress, Appraisal and Coping*. New York: Springer.

Lea, A. (1994) Defining the roles of lay and nursing caring. *Nursing Standard*, **9**, 5, 32-35.

Lees, S.D. and Lepage, P. (1994) Will robots ever replace attendants? Explaining the current capabilities and future potential of robots in education and rehabilitation. *International Journal of Rehabilitation Research*, **17**, 285-304.

Lefebvre, C. (1994) The Cochrane Collaboration: the role of the UK Cochrane Centre in identifying the evidence. *Health Libraries Review*, **11**, 235-242.

Leidy, N.K., Ozbolt, J.G., Swain, M.A.P. (1990) Psycho-physiological process of stress in chronic physical illness: a theoretical perspective. *Journal of Advanced Nursing*, **15**, 478-486.

Lenz, E.R., Supre, F., Gift, A.G. et al (1995) Collaborative development of middle-range nursing theories: toward a theory of unpleasant symptoms. *Advances in Nursing Science*, **17**, 3, 1-13.

Levine, M.E. (1995) The rhetoric of nursing theory. *Image*, **27**, 1, 11-14.

Lewin, B. (1995) Psychological factors in cardiac rehabilitation. In: Jones, D. and West, R. (Eds) *Cardiac Rehabilitation*. London: BMJ Publishing Group.

Lewinter, M. and Mikkelsen, S. (1995a) Patients' experience of rehabilitation after stroke. *Disability and Rehabilitation*, **17**, 1, 3-9.

Lewinter, M. and Mikkelsen, S. (1995b) Therapists and the rehabilitation process after a stroke. *Disability and Rehabilitation*, **17**, 5, 211-216.

Lewis, J. and Meredith, B. (1988a) *Daughters Who Care: Daughters caring for mothers at home*. London: Routledge and Kegan Paul.

Lewis, J. and Meredith, B. (1988b) Daughters caring for mothers. *Ageing and Society*, **8**, 1, 1-21.

Lindgren, C.L., Burke, M.L., Hainsworth, M.A., Eakes, G.G. (1992) Chronic sorrow: a life-span concept. *Scholarly Inquiry for Nursing Practice*, **6**, 27-42.

Lindsey, E. (1996) Health within illness: experiences of chronically ill/disabled people. *Journal of Advanced Nursing*, **24**, 3, 465-472.

Livneh, H. (1995) The tripartite model of rehabilitation interventions: basics, goals and rehabilitation strategies. *Journal of Applied Rehabilitation Counselling*, **26**, 1, 25-29.

Loveys, B. (1990) Transition in chronic illness: the at risk role. *Holistic Nursing Practice*, **4**, 3, 56-64.

Luborsky, M.R. (1995) The process of self report of impairment in clinical research. *Social Science and Medicine*, **40**, 11, 1447-1459.

Lyons, R.F., Sullivan, M.J.L., Ritvo, P.G., Coyne, J.C. (1995) *Relationships in Chronic Illness and Disability*. Thousand Oakes, California: Sage.

Malan, S.S. (1992) Psychosocial adjustment following MI: current views and nursing implications. *Journal of Cardiovascular Nursing*, **6**, 57-70.

Marris, V. (1996) *Lives Worth Living: Women's experience of chronic illness*. London: Pandora.

Martin, S.D. (1995) Coping with chronic illness. *Home Healthcare Nurse*, **13**, 4, 50-54.

Masterson, A. (1994) Disability. In: Gough, P., Maslin-Prothero, S., Masterson, A. (Eds) *Nursing and Social Policy: Care in context*. London: Butterworth Heinnemann.

McBride, A.B. (1993) Managing chronicity. The heart of nursing care. In: Funk, S.G., Tornquist, E.M.T., Champagne, S.T., Wiese R A (Eds) *Key Aspects of Elder Care: Managing falls, incontinence and cognitive impairment*. New York: Springer.

McCormick, L. and Goldman, R. (1979) The transdisciplinary model: implications for service delivery and personnel preparation for the severely and profoundly handicapped. *ASESPH Review*, **4**, 2, 152-161.

McCoy, P. (1983) Short-term residential care for older people: an answer to growing older. In: Jerrome, D. (Ed.) *Ageing in Modern Society*. London: Croom Helm.

References

McDaniel, R.W. and Bach, C.A. (1994) Quality of life: a concept analysis. *Rehabilitation Nursing Research*, **3**, 18-22.

McFall, R.M. (1993) The essential role of theory in psychological assessment. In: Gluekauf, R.L., Sechrest, L.B., Bond. G.R., McDaniel, E.G. (Ed.) *Improving Assessment in Rehabilitation and Health*. Newbury Park: Sage.

McGrath, M. (1991) *Multidisciplinary Teamwork*. Aldershot: Avebury.

McKee, K.J. (1994) *Coping in Family Carers of Elderly People with Dementia*. Paper presented at the Alzheimer's disease Tenth International Conference, Edinburgh.

McLaughlin, J. and Zeeberg, I. (1993) Self-care and multiple-sclerosis – a view from 2 cultures. *Social Science and Medicine*, **37**, 315-329.

Mechanic, D. (1995a) Sociological dimensions of illness behaviour. *Social Science Medicine*, **41**(a), 1267-1216.

Mechanic, D. (1995b) Emerging trends in the application and social sciences to health and medicine. *Social Science and Medicine*, **11**, 1491-1496.

Melvin, J.L (1989) Status report on interdisciplinary medical rehabilitation. *Archives of Physical Medicine and Rehabilitation*, **70**, 273-276.

Metcalfe, S.A. (1995) Disability: a patient's perspective on rehabilitation. *British Journal of Therapy and Rehabilitation*, **2**, 2, 57-58.

Miller, J.F. (1992a) Patient power resources. In: Miller, J.F. (Ed.) *Coping with Chronic Illness: Overcoming powerlessness* (2nd Edn). Philadelphia: FA Davies.

Miller, J.F. (1992b) Concept development of powerlessness: a nursing diagnosis. In: Miller, J.F. (Ed.) *Coping with Chronic Illness: Overcoming powerlessness* (2nd Edn). Philadelphia: FA Davies.

Miller, J.F. (1992c) Analysis of coping with illness. In: Miller, J.F. (Ed.) *Coping with Chronic Illness: Overcoming powerlessness* (2nd Edn). Philadelphia: FA Davies.

Miller, J.F. (1992d) Enabling self esteem. In: Miller, J.F. (Ed.) *Coping with Chronic Illness: Overcoming powerlessness* (2nd Edn). Philadelphia: FA Davies.

Miller, J.F. (1992e) Inspiring hope. In: Miller, J.F. (Ed.) *Coping with Chronic Illness: Overcoming powerlessness* (2nd Edn). Philadelphia: FA Davies.

Milz, M. (1992) Healthy ill people: social cynicism or new perspectives. In: Kaplun, A. (Ed.) *Health Promotion and Chronic Illness: Discovering a new quality of health*. Copenhagen: WHO Regional Publication, European Series No. 44.

Mishel, M.H. and Braden, C.J. (1988) Finding meaning: antecedents of uncertainty in illness. *Nursing Research*, **37**, 2, 98-103, 127.

Mishel, M.H. (1993) Living with chronic illness: living with uncertainty. In: Funk, S.G., Tornquist, E.M.T., Champagne, S.T., Wiese, R.A. (Eds) *Key Aspects of Elder Care: Managing falls, incontinence and cognitive impairment*. New York: Springer.

Morse, J.M. (1994) Emerging from the data: the cognitive processes of analysis in qualitative inquiry. In: Morse, J.M. (Ed.) *Critical Issues in Qualitative Research Methods*. Thousand Oaks: Sage.

Morse, J.M. and Doberneck, B. (1995) Delineating the concept of hope. *Image: Journal of Nursing Scholarship*, **27**, 4, 277-285.

Morse, J.M. and Johnson, J.L. (1991) Towards a theory of illness: the illness constellation model. In: Morse, J.M. and Johnson, J.L. (Eds) *The Illness Experience: Dimensions of suffering*. Newbury Park: Sage.

Morse, J.M. and O'Brien, B. (1995) Preserving self from victim to patient to disabled person. *Journal of Advanced Nursing*, **21**, 5, 886-896.

Moss-Morris, R. and Petrie, K. (1994) Illness perceptions: implications for occupational therapy. *Australian Occupational Therapy Journal*, **41**, 2, 73-82.

Mosqueda, L.A. (1993) Assessment of rehabilitation potential. *Clinics in Geriatric Medicine*, **9**, 4, 689-703.

Mulley, G.P. (1994) Principles of rehabilitation. *Reviews in Clinical Gerontology*, **4**, 61-69.

Mullins, L.L. (1989) Hate revisited: power, envy and greed in the rehabilitation setting. *Archives of Physical and Medical Rehabilitation*, **70**, 740-744.

Mumma, C.M. and Nelson, A. (1996) Models for theory based practice of rehabilitation nursing. In: Hoeman, S.P. (1996) *Rehabilitation Nursing: Process and application* (2nd Edn). St Louis: Mosby.

Myco, F. (1984) Stroke and its rehabilitation: the perceived role of the nurse in medical and nursing literature. *Journal of Advanced Nursing*, **9**, 429-439.

National Opinion Poll (1996) *Disability and rehabilitation projects: Phase I.* London: Qualitative Study, NOP.

Neal, L.J. (1995) The rehabilitation nursing team in the home health care setting. *Rehabilitation Nursing*, **20**, 1, 32-36.

NHS Centre for Reviews and Dissemination (1996) *Undertaking Literature Reviews of Research on Effectiveness: CRD guidelines for those carrying out or commissioning reviews.* ORD Report 4. York: University of York.

Nolan, M.R. (1992) Developing a 'seamless service': future reality or new policy rhetoric? *BASELINE*, **49**, 21-28.

Nolan, M.R. and Grant, G. (1992a) *Regular Respite: An evaluation of a hospital rota bed scheme for elderly people.* London: Age Concern.

Nolan, M.R. and Grant, G. (1992b) Helping new carers of the frail elderly patient: the challenge for nursing in acute care settings. *Journal of Clinical Nursing*, **1**, 303-307.

Nolan, M.R. and Grant, G. (1994) Mid-range theory building and the theory-practice gap: a respite care case study. In: Smith, J.P. (Ed.) *Models, Theories and Concepts.* Oxford: Blackwell Scientific Publishers.

Nolan, M.R., Grant, G., Caldock, K., Keady, J. (1994) *A Framework for Assessing the Needs of Family Carers: A multi-disciplinary guide.* Stoke-on-Trent: BASE Publications.

Nolan, M.R., Grant, G., Nolan, J. (1995) Busy doing nothing: activity and interaction levels amongst differing populations of elderly patients. *Journal of Advanced Nursing*, **22**, 3, 528-538.

Nolan, M.R., Grant, G., Keady, J. (1996) *Understanding Family Care: A multidimensional model of caring and coping.* Buckingham: Open University Press.

Nolan, M.R., Nolan, J., Booth, A. (1997) *Preparing for Multi-professional/Multi-agency Health Care Practice: The nursing contribution to rehabilitation within the multi-disciplinary team. Literature review and curriculum analysis.* Final Report to English National Board for Nursing, Midwifery and Health Visiting.

Nordstrom, M.J. (1980) Criteria leading to quality control in rehabilitation: the elderly patient – a team member. *Journal of Geriatric Nursing*, **6**, 8, 457-462.

O'Connor, S.E. (1993) Nursing and rehabilitation: the interventions of nurses in stroke. *Journal of Clinical Nursing*, **2**, 29-34.

Oliver, M. (1986) Social policy and disability: some theoretical issues. *Disability, Handicap and Society*, **1**, 1, 5-17.

Oliver, M., Zarb, G., Silver, S., Moore, M., Salisburg, V. (1988) *Walking into Darkness: The experience of spinal cord injury.* Basingstoke: Macmillan.

Oliver, M. (1990) *The Politics of Disablement.* Basingstoke: Macmillan.

Oliver, M. (1993) A different viewpoint – who needs rehabilitating? In: Greenwood, R., Barnes, M.P., McMillan, T.M., Ward, C.D. (Eds) *Neurological Rehabilitation.* Edinburgh: Churchill Livingstone.

Ottenbacher, K.J. (1990) Clinically relevant design for rehabilitation: the idiographic model. *American Journal of Physical Medicine and Rehabilitation*, **69**, 6, 286-292.

Øvretveit, J. (1990) Making the team work. *Professional Nurse*, **5**, 6, 284-288.

Øvretveit, J. (1993) *Coordinating Community Care: Multidisciplinary teamwork and care management.* Buckingham: Open University Press.

Oxman, A.S. (1994) *Section VI: Preparing and maintaining systematic reviews. The Cochrane Collaboration Handbook.* Oxford: Cochrane Collaboration.

Palat, M. (1992) The triangulation model of rehabilitation medicine. *European Rehabilitation*, **2**, 85-87.

Partridge, C.J. (1980) The effectiveness of physiotherapy: a classification for evaluation. *Physiotherapy*, **66**, 153-155.

Partridge, C. and Johnston, M. (1989) Perceived context of recovery from physical disability: measurement and prediction. *British Journal of Clinical Psychology*, **28**, 53-59.

Paul, R.W. and Heaslip, P. (1995) Critical thinking and intuitive nursing practice. *Journal of Advanced Nursing*, **22**, 1, 40-47.

References

Pawlson, L.G. (1994) Health care reform. Chronic illness – implications of a new paradigm for health care. *Joint Commission Journal on Quality Improvement*, **20**, 1, 33-39.

Peace, G. (1996) Living under the shadow of illness. *Nursing Times*, **92**, 28, 46-48.

Pearlin, L.I. and Scholler, C. (1978) The structure of coping. *Journal of Health and Social Behaviour*, **19**, 12-21.

Peplau, H.E. (1995) Foreword ix-x. In: Farran, C.J., Keith, K.A., Popovich, J.M. (Eds) *Hope and Hopelessness: Critical clinical constructs*. Thousand Oakes, California: Sage.

Perry, E. (1991) Living with rheumatoid arthritis. *Nursing Times*, **87**, 58-60.

Peters, D.J. (1995) Human experience in disablement: the impetus of the ICIDH. *Disability and Rehabilitation*, **17**, 214, 135-144.

Philp, I. (1996) Comment: community alternatives to hospital care. *Reviews in Clinical Gerontology*, **6**, 195-196.

Pitkeathley, J. (1990) Painful conflicts. *Community Care (Inside)*, 802, 22 February, i-ii.

Pollock, S.E. (1993) Adaptations to chronic illness: a program of research for testing nursing theory. *Nursing Science Quarterly*, **6**, 2, 86-92.

Pollock, C., Freemandle, N., Sheldon, T. et al (1993) Methodological difficulties in rehabilitation research. *Clinical Rehabilitation*, 7, 63-72.

Porter, E.J. (1995) A phenomenological alternative to the 'ADL research tradition'. *Journal of Aging and Health*, 7, 1, 24-45.

Pott, E. (1992) Preface xi-xv. In: Kaplun, A. (Ed.) *Health Promotion and Chronic Illness: Discovering a new quality of health*. Copenhagen: WHO Regional Publications, European Series No. 44.

Pound, P., Bury, M., Gompertz, P., Ebrahim, S. (1995) Stroke patients' views on their admission to hospital. *British Medical Journal*, **311**, 1 July, 18-22.

Preston, K. (1994) Rehabilitation nursing: a client centred philosophy. *American Journal of Nursing*, **94**, 2, February 1994, 66-70.

Price, M.J. (1993) Exploration of body listening: health and physical self-awareness in chronic illness. *Advances in Nursing Science*, **15**, 37-52.

Price, B. (1996) Illness careers: the chronic illness experience. *Journal of Advanced Nursing*, **24**, 2, 275-279.

Purk, J.K. (1993) Rehabilitation staff nurses' job satisfaction. *Rehabilitation Nursing*, **18**, 4, 249-252.

Qualls, S.H. and Czirr, R. (1988) Geriatric health teams: clarifying models of professional and team functioning. *The Gerontologist*, **28**, 3, 372-376.

Quinn, A.A., Barton, J.A., Magilvy, J.K. (1995) Weathering the storm: metaphors and stories of living with multiple sclerosis. *Rehabilitation Nursing Research*, **4**, 19-27.

Radley, A. (1994) *Making Sense of Illness: The social psychology of health and disease*. London: Sage.

Radley, A. and Green, R. (1987) Illness as adjustment: a methodology and conceptual framework. *Society of Health and Illness*, **9**, 2, 179-207.

Raeburn, J.M. and Rootman, I. (1996) Quality of life and health promotion. In: Renwick, R., Brown, I., Nagler, M. (Eds) *Quality of Life in Health Promotion and Rehabilitation: Conceptual approaches, issues and applications*. Thousand Oakes, California: Sage.

Ragnarsson, K.T. and Gordon, W.A. (1992) Rehabilitation after spinal cord injury: the team approach. *Physical Medicine and Rehabilitation Clinics of North America*, **3**, 853-878.

Renwick, R. and Brown, I. (1996) The centre for health practitioners: conceptual approach to quality of life, being, belonging and becoming. In: Renwick, R., Brown, I., Nagler, M. (Eds) *Quality of Life in Health Promotion and Rehabilitation: Conceptual approaches, issues and applications*. Thousand Oakes, California: Sage.

Renwick, R, and Friefield, S. (1996) Quality of life and rehabilitation. In: Renwick, R., Brown, I., Nagler, M. (Eds) *Quality of Life in Health Promotion and Rehabilitation: Conceptual approaches, issues and applications*. Thousand Oakes, California: Sage.

Renwick, R., Brown, I. Nagler, M. (1996) (Eds) *Quality of Life in Health Promotion and Rehabilitation: Conceptual approaches, issues and applications*. Thousand Oakes, California: Sage.

Resnick, B. (1996) Motivation in geriatric rehabilitation. *Image*, **28**, 1, 41-45.

Rieve, J.E. (1989) Sexuality and the adult with acquired physical disability. *Nursing Clinics of North America*, **24**, 1, 265-276.

Ricke, A. (1992) Medical training: a serious deficit. In: Kaplun, A. (Ed.) *Health Promotion and Chronic Illness: Discovering a new quality of health.* Copenhagen: WHO Regional Publications, European Series No. 44.

Rijke, R.P.C. and Rijke-de-Vries, J. (1992) Health promotion for health professionals. In: Kaplun, A. (Ed.) *Health Promotion and Chronic Illness: Discovering a new quality of health.* Copenhagen: WHO Regional Publications, European Series No. 44.

Robinson, I. (1988) The rehabilitation of patients with long term physical impairments: the social context of professional roles. *Clinical Rehabilitation,* **2**, 339-347.

Robinson, I. (1989) Reconstructing lives: negotiating the meaning of multiple sclerosis. In: Robinson, I. and Bury, M. (Eds) *Living with Chronic Illness.* Cambridge: Cambridge University Press.

Robinson, I. (1990) Personal narratives, social careers and medical courses – analyzing life trajectories in autobiographies of people with multiple sclerosis. *Social Science and Medicine,* **30**, 1173-1186.

Robinson, C.A. (1995) Unifying distinctions for nursing research with persons and families. *Journal of Family Nursing,* **1**, 1, 8-29.

Robinson, L.A., Bevil, C., Arcangelo, V. et al (1993) Operationalising the Corbin and Strauss Trajectory Model for elderly clients with chronic illness. *Scholarly Inquiry for Nursing Practice,* 7, 4, 253-264.

Robinson, J. and Batstone, G. (1996) *Rehabilitation: A development challenge.* King's Fund Working Paper. London: King's Fund.

Rolland, J.S. (1988) A conceptual model of chronic and life threatening illness and its impact on families. In: Chilman, C.S., Nunnally, E.W., Cox, F.M. (Eds) *Chronic Illness and Disabilities.* Beverly Hills, Sage.

Rolland, J.S. (1990) Anticipating loss: a family systems development framework. *Family Process,* **29**, 3, 229-244.

Rolland, J.S. (1994) *Families, Illness and Disability: An integrative treatment model.* New York: Basic Books.

Rossiter, D. and Thompson, A.J. (1995) Introduction of integrated care pathways for patients with multiple sclerosis in any inpatient neuro-rehabilitation setting. *Disability and Rehabilitation,* **17**, 8, 443-448.

Rothberg, J.S. (1981) The rehabilitation team – future direction. *Archives of Physical Medicine and Rehabilitation,* **62**, 407-410.

Rowbottom, J. (1992) *Seamless Service: A stitch in time – care in the community.* Occasional Paper No. 1. London: Institute of Health Services Management.

Royal College of Nursing (1994) *Standards of Care: Rehabilitation nursing.* Rehabilitation Nurses Forum Committee. London: RCN.

Royal College of Nursing (1996) *The Value and Skills of Nurses Working with Older People.* London: RCN.

Royal College of Physicians (1986) Physical disability in 1986 and beyond. *Journal of Royal College of Physicians,* **20**, 3, 160-194.

Ryan, P. (1992) Facilitating behaviour: change in the chronically ill. In: Miller, J.F. (Ed.) *Coping with Chronic Illness: Overcoming powerlessness* (2nd Edn). Philadelphia: FA Davies.

Schaefer, K.M. (1995) Women living in paradox: loss and discovery in chronic illness. *Holistic Nursing Practice,* **9**, 3, 63-74.

Schut, H.A. and Stam, H.J. (1994) Goals in rehabilitation teamwork. *Disability and Rehabilitation,* **16**, 4, 223-226.

Schultz, R. and Williamson, G.M. (1993) Psychosocial and behavioural dimensions of physical frailty. *Journal of Gerontology,* **48**, (special edition), 39-43.

Schussler, G. (1992) Coping strategies and individual meaning of illness. *Social Science and Medicine,* **34**, 4, 427-432.

Scullion, P. (1995) Disability research and health care professionals: some issues for debate. *British Journal of Therapy and Rehabilitation,* **2**, 6, 318-322.

Secretary of State for Health (1996a) *The National Health Service: A service with ambitions* CM3425. London: The Stationery Office.

References   Secretary of State for Health (1996b) *Primary Care: The future choice and opportunity*. London: The Stationery Office.

Secretary of State for Health (1996c) *Primary Care: Delivering the future*. London: The Stationery Office.

Shaw, M.C. and Halliday, P.H. (1992) The family, crises and chronic illness: an evolutionary model. *Journal of Advanced Nursing*, 17, 537-543.

Sheppard, B. (1994a) *Listening to patients: An action research project*. Brighton: Brighton Health Care NHS Trust.

Sheppard, B. (1994b) *Looking Back, Moving Forward: Developing elderly care, rehabilitation and the nurse's role within it*. Brighton: Brighton Health Care NHS Trust.

Siegrist, S. (1995) Social differential in chronic disease: what could sociological knowledge offer to explain and possibly relieve illness? (Editorial). *Social Science Medicine*, 41, 12, 1603-1605.

SNMAC (1995) *In the Patient's Interest: Multi-professional working across organisation boundaries*. London: DoH.

Soeken, K.L. and Carson, V.J. (1987) Responding to the spiritual needs of the chronically ill. *Nursing Clinics in North America*, 22, 3, 603-611.

Spencer, J., Young, M.E., Rintala, D., Bates, S. (1995) Socialisation to the culture of a rehabilitation hospital. an ethnographic study. *The American Journal of Occupational Therapy*, 29, 1, 35-62.

Spoltore, T.A. and O'Brien, A.M. (1995) Rehabilitation of the spinal cord. *Orthopaedic Nursing*, 14, 3, 7-14.

Squires, A.J. (1996) Overview and future of rehabilitation of older people. In: Squires, A.J. (Ed.) *Rehabilitation of Older People: A handbook for the MDT* (2nd Edn). London: Chapman Hall.

Stapleton, S. (1992) Decreasing powerlessness in the chronically ill: a prototypical plan. In: Miller, J.F. (Ed.) *Coping with Chronic Illness: Overcoming powerlessness* (2nd Edn). Philadelphia: FA Davies.

Stephens, R. (1992) Imagery as a means in coping. In: Miller, J.F. (Ed.) *Coping with Chronic Illness: Overcoming powerlessness* (2nd Edn). Philadelphia: FA Davies.

Stewart, B.J., Archbold, P.G., Harvath, T.A., Nkongho, N.O. (1993) Role acquisition in family caregivers of older people who have been discharged from hospital. In: Funk, S.G., Tornquist, E.H., Champagne, M.T., Weise, R.A. (Eds) *Key Aspects of Caring for the Chronically Ill: Hospital and home*. New York: Springer.

Stetz, K.M., Lewis, F.M., Houck, G.M. (1994) Family goals, an indication of adaptation during chronic illness. *Public Health Nursing*, 11, 6, 385-391.

Stoller, E.P. and Pugliesi, K.L. (1989) Other roles of caregivers: competing responsibilities or supportive resources? *Journal of Gerontology (Social Services)*, 44, 6, 5, 231-232.

Strauss, A.L., Corbin, J.M., Fagerhaugh, S. et al (1984) *Chronic Illness and the Quality of Life* (2nd Edn). St Louis: Mosby.

Strauss, A.L. and Corbin, J.M. (1988) *Shaping a New Health Care System: The experience of chronic illness as a catalyst for change*. San Francisco: Jossey-Bass.

Stryker, R. (1996) Foreword xvii. In: Hoeman, S.P. (Ed.) *Rehabilitation Nursing: Process and application* (2nd Edn). St Louis: Mosby.

Studenski, S. and Duncan, P.W. (1993) Measuring rehabilitation outcomes: geriatric rehabilitation. *Clinics in Geriatric Medicine*, 9, 11, 823-830.

Sundance, P. and Cope, D.N. (1995) Outcome Level 1, physiologic stability – acute management. In: Landrum, P.K., Schmidt, N.D., McLean, A. Jr (Eds) *Outcome Orientated Rehabilitation: Principles, strategies and tools for effective program management*. Gaithenburg: Aspen Publications.

Swift, C. (1989) Health care of the elderly: the concept of progress. In: Warnes, A.M. (Ed.) *Human Ageing and Later Life: Multidisciplinary perspectives*. London: Edward Arnold.

Swift, C.G. (1996) Disease and disability in older people: prospects for intervention. In: Squires, A.J. (Ed.) *Rehabilitation of Older People: A handbook for the MDT* (2nd Edn). London: Chapman Hall.

Symington, D.C. (1994) Megatrends in rehabilitation: a Canadian perspective. *International Journal of Rehabilitation Research*, 17, 1-14.

Tallis, R. (1989) Measurement and future of rehabilitation. *Geriatric Medicine*, 19, 1, 31-40.

Tallis, R. (1992) Rehabilitation of the elderly in the 21st century. *Journal of the Royal College of Physicians*, **26**, 4, 413-422.

Talo, S., Rytökoski, U., Puukka, R., Alanen, E. et al (1995) An experimental investigation of the biopsychosocial disease consequence model: psychological implications, disability and handicap in chronic pain patients. *Disability and Rehabilitation*, **17**, 6, 281-292.

Taraborrelli, P. (1993) Exemplar A: becoming a carer. In: Gilbert, N. (Ed.) *Researching Social Life*. London: Sage.

Thompson, P. (1992) I don't feel old: subjective ageing and the search for meaning in life. *Ageing and Society*, **12**, 23-47.

Thompson, S.C. and Pitts, J.S. (1992) In sickness and in health: chronic illness, marriage and spousal caregiving. In: Spacapan, S. and Oskamp, S. (Eds) *Helping and Being Helped: Naturalistic studies*. Newbury Park: Sage.

Thompson, D.R., Ersser, S.J., Webster, R.A. (1995) The experiences of patients and their partners 1 month after a heart attack. *Journal of Advanced Nursing*, **22**, 707-714.

Thorne, S.E. (1993) *Negotiating Health Care: The social context of chronic illness*. Newbury Park: Sage.

Thurgood, A. (1990) Seven steps to rehabilitation. *Nursing Times*, **86**, 25, 38-41.

Toombs, S.K., Barnard, D., Carson, R.A. (1995) *Chronic Illness: From experience to policy*. Bloomington: Indiana University Press.

Tranter, R.T., Slater, R., Vaughan, N. (1995) Physically disabled and frail elders: assessing their external environments. *Disability and Rehabilitation*, **17**, 305-311.

Trexler, L.E. and Fordyce, D.J. (1996) Psychological perspectives on rehabilitation: contemporary assessment and intervention strategies. In: Bushbacher, R.M., Dimitru, D., Johnson, E.W. (Eds) *Physical Medicine and Rehabilitation*. Philadelphia: Saunders.

Trieschmann, R.B. (1995) The energy model: a new approach to rehabilitation. *Rehabilitation Education*, **9**, 2, 217-227.

Turnbull, A.P. and Turnbull, H.R. (1993) Participatory research in cognitive coping: from concepts to research planning. In: Turnbull, A.P., Patterson, J.M., Behr, S.K. et al (Eds) *Cognitive Coping, Families and Disability*. Baltimore: Paul H Brookes.

Twigg, J. and Atkin, K. (1994) *Carers Perceived: Policy and practice in informal care*. Buckingham: Open University Press.

Twinning, C. (1996) Psychological approaches with older people. In: Squires, A.J. (Ed.) *Rehabilitation of Older People: A handbook for the MDT* (2nd Edn). London: Chapman Hall.

Van Bennekom C.A.M., Jelles, F., Lankhorst, G.J. (1995) Rehabilitation activities profile: the ICIDH as a framework for a problem-orientated assessment method in rehabilitation medicine. *Disability and Rehabilitation*, **17**, 314, 169-175.

Vaughan, C. and Bhakta, B. (1995) Recent advances in rehabilitation medicine. *Journal of the Royal College of Physicians of London*, **29**, 6, 534-539.

Verbrugge, L.M. and Jette, A.M. (1994) The disablement process. *Social Science and Medicine*, **38**, 1, 1-14.

Ville, I., Ravaud, J.F., Diard, C., Paicheler, H. (1994) Self representations and physical impairment: a social constructionalist approach. *Society of Health and Illness*, **16**, 3, 301-321.

Vreede, C.F. (1988) The need for a better definition of activities of daily living. *International Journal of Rehabilitation Research*, **11**, 1, 29-35.

Walker, G. (1995) Therapists and nurses in older people's rehabilitation: unmet role performance expectations. *British Journal of Therapy and Rehabilitation*, **2**, 1, 9-12.

Walley, H.M.L. (1986) *Ward Sister's Concept of Rehabilitation*. Unpublished MSc Dissertation, University of Southampton.

Ward, C.D. and McIntosh, S. (1993) The rehabilitation process: a neurological perspective. In: Greenwood, R., Barnes, M.P., McMillan, T.M., Ward, C.D. (Eds) *Neurological Nursing*. Edinburgh: Churchill Livingstone.

Waters, K.R. (1987) The role of nursing in rehabilitation care. *Science and Practice*, **5**, 3, 17-21.

Waters, K.R. (1991) *The Role of the Nurse in Rehabilitation of Elderly People in Hospital*. Unpublished PhD Thesis, University of Manchester.

References   Waters, K.R. (1996) Rehabilitation: core themes in gerontological nursing. In: Wade, L. and Waters, K.R. (Eds) *A Textbook of Gerontological Nursing: Perspectives on practice.* London: Baillière Tindall.

Waters, K.R. and Luker, K.A. (1996) Staff perspectives on the role of the nurse in rehabilitation wards for elderly people. *Journal of Clinical Nursing*, **5**, 2, 103-114.

Weeks, S.K. and O'Connor P.C. (1994) Concept analysis of family and health: a new definition of family health. *Rehabilitation Nursing*, **19**, 4, 207-210.

Weinberger, M., Tierney, W.M., Booher, P., Hiner, L. (1990) Social support: stress and functional status with osteoarthritis. *Social Science and Medicine*, **30**, 4, 503-508.

Wells, T.J. (1980) *Problems in Geriatric Nursing.* Edinburgh: Churchill Livingstone.

Whalley-Hammell, K.R.W. (1992) Psychological and sociological theories concerning adjustment to traumatic spinal cord injury – the implications for rehabilitation. *Paraplegia*, **30**, 317-326.

Whalley-Hammell, K.W. (1995) Spinal cord injury; quality of life; occupational therapy: is there a connection? *British Journal of Occupational Therapy*, **58**, 151-157.

Wild, D. (1994) Stroke: a nursing rehabilitation role. *Nursing Standard*, **8**, 17, 36-39.

Wilkin, D. and Hughes, B. (1986) The elderly and the health services. In: Phillipson, C. and Walker, A. (Eds) *Ageing and Social Policy: A continual assessment.* Aldershot: Gower.

Williams, G. (1984) The genesis of chronic illness – narrative re-construction. *Sociology of Health and Illness*, **6**, 175-200.

Williams, G.H. and Wood, P.H. (1988) Coming to terms with chronic illness: the negotiation of autonomy in rheumatoid arthritis. *International Journal of Disability Studies*, **10**, 128-133.

Williams, J. (1994) The rehabilitation process for older people and their carers. *Nursing Times*, **90**, 29, 33-34.

Williamson, C. (1992) *Whose Standards? Consumer and professional standards in health care.* Buckingham: Open University Press.

Wistow, G. (1995) Aspirations and realities: community care at the crossroads. *Health and Social Care in the Community*, **3**, 4, 227-240.

Wood, R.W. (1993) The rehabilitation team. In: Greenwood, R., Barnes, M.P., McMillan, T.M., Ward C.D. (Eds) *Neurological Rehabilitation.* Edinburgh: Churchill Livingstone.

Woods, N.F., Hoberman, M.R., Packard, N.J. (1993) Demands of illness and individual dyadic and family adaptations in chronic illness. *Journal of Nursing Research*, **15**, 1, 10-25.

Woods, N.F. and Lewis, F.M. (1995) Women with chronic illness: their views of their families' adaptation. *Health Care for Women International*, **16**, 135-148.

Woog, P. (1992) *The Chronic Illness Trajectory Framework: The Corbin and Strauss nursing model.* New York: Springer.

World Health Organisation (1980) *International Classification of Impairments, Disabilities and Handicaps: A manual of classification relating to the consequence of disease.* Geneva: WHO.

Worthington, J. (1994) Team approach to multidisciplinary care. *British Journal of Therapy and Rehabilitation*, **1**, 314, 119-120.

Yoshida, K.K. (1993) Reshaping of self: a pendular reconstruction of self and identity among adults with traumatic spinal cord injury. *Sociology of Health and Illness*, **15**, 2, 217-245.

Yoshida, K.K. (1994) Institutional impact on self concept among persons with spinal cord injury. *International Journal of Rehabilitation Research*, **17**, 95-107.

Young, J.B. (1995) Black families with a chronically disabled family member: a framework for study. *The ABNF Journal*, **6**, 3, 68-73.

Young, J.B. and Gladman, J.R.F. (1995) Future directions in stroke rehabilitation. *Reviews in Clinical Gerontology*, **5**, 329-337.